The Multi-Generational Poisoning of America:

If You Want the Truth, Ask This Nurse . . .

By

Geraldine Fiedler

AF882741

First printing.

Published by
Vanderblumen Publications
P.O. Box 626
La Mesa, CA 91944

Softcover: ISBN: 978-0-615-59190-2

La Mesa, California

Printed in the United State of America

Dedication

FOR ALL HUMANITY
PAST, PRESENT, AND FUTURE

Acknowledgements

To my family and friends who helped me through the horrible experiences I describe here.

To the physicians and nurses at Mercy Hospital who provided the guidance, support and courage to know and tell the truth about chemicals and pesticides.

To the Nuns, the actual Angels of Mercy Hospital, who provided the spiritual guidance in the healing professions.

This work would not have been possible without the hard work of my researcher, copyeditor and typist, Jo Cryder. Her research and organizational skills are a true contribution and benefit to this work.

Special thanks to my consulting publisher and editor, Glenna Bloemen. Without her hours of work to produce this publication, the truth may never have seen the light of day.

TABLE OF CONTENTS

INTRODUCTION

Nurses are the listeners and problem solvers of our society. They are always ready to help anyone and they deserve more credit for their efforts then they are currently receiving. In 1959, I saw the dangers of chemical exposure having first-hand experience. Having survive this experience, this has become my purpose in life to get the word out about the harmful effects of pesticides and chemicals.

I am only one person and I cannot do it alone. I tried by suing the local pest control company that placed DDT directly inside the closet of my home. This exposure resulted in severe illness from which I was lucky to have survived. I lost my case, but not my voice. This is my story and this is my message.

All parents and grandparents must demand that the multi-generational poisoning of our food, water, and air be stopped immediately. It may be too late for my generation, but we must do it for the next generations, our children and grandchildren! Parents often come to me often asking for answers to questions about the health of their children and grandchildren.

Mankind is polluting himself out of existence and all for money! Money is the root of this evil. For your children's' sake, pediatricians should be telling you to avoid chemicals in foods and all pesticides in your environment.

As early as 1960, Dr. Francis Pottenger and Senator Samuel Geddes said, "Man will pollute himself out of existence." It has happened and will continue to happen unless we do something about it.

Recently in San Diego, California, 1,500 children demonstrated in Balboa Park carrying signs that read, "Stop the Poisoning." They're not alone. I did a search on the internet under "Stop the Poisoning" and I found 67,800 results. Are you listening? The sicker all of us are, the more money the medical establishment makes, the more the pesticide and chemical companies make, and the more our loved ones get sick and die.

In the 1950's, I was a human guinea pig. We know firsthand how my family and I were poisoned by DDT. As a result of that experience, I tried to stop the insane spraying of schoolyards and students in classrooms in the 50's and 60's. I knew then how dangerous pesticides and chemicals were and still are.

In 1959, my family was poisoned by a commercial concentration of 50 percent **DDT**. The **DDT** was applied as a powder dust in our bedroom closet and through the ventilating system was blown throughout our house.

For years we have all been fooled by the pesticide and chemical companies and their claims that their compounds only kill bugs and do not damage or kill adults or our children. I believe this to be the fatal cover-up that we see in the television commercials. Don't believe them. Pesticides and chemicals and their misuse have contaminated our planet.

As a result, today we have diseases that I never heard of as a registered nurse with over 70 years of experience. For instance, the escalation of autism in children has risen significantly.

According to the findings of the Autism Research Institute, "the prevalence of autism is about 1-2 per 1,000 people; the prevalence of **ASD** is about 6 per 1,000, with about four times as many males as females. The number of people diagnosed with autism has increased dramatically since the 1980s, partly due to changes in diagnostic practice; the question of whether actual prevalence has increased is unresolved."

For further information, read the footnotes and references are located in the back of this book.

My best friend, Jean Neisewander, has one grandchild who is autistic. Could pesticides have caused his **autism**? Some scientists believe so.

This is my story. I want the public to realize how serious this issue has become. The harmful effects of the use and misuse of pesticides and chemicals have altered the course of our civilization and not always for the better.

In our attempts to improve our food sources, we have caused disease to increase. We did not know then what the consequences would be from our actions. However, we know now and it is time to stop.

Chapter One
I Was A DDT Cripple

My purpose in recounting my experiences with insecticide poisoning is to provide a first-hand account of the little recognized effects of such poisoning in order to alert the medical profession and the American public of this menace to health.

Additionally, I am suggesting areas I believe to be related to poisoning that need to be thoroughly investigated, such as crib death, food contamination, and exposure of school children and contamination of household furnishings. My training as a registered nurse has enabled me to report symptoms objectively as well as to bridge the gap between consumer and the medical profession.

In 1959, I had my home sprayed by a local pest control company for a few Oriental roaches that had entered my bedroom closet. At first, we noticed no adverse effects from this spray and the family appeared to remain in good health.

However, since the **Diazinon** they used did not kill the roaches, I again called the pest control company. This time the pest control operator threw a white powder into the small built-in storage area which was within the bedroom closet itself. He did not say exactly what this powder was, but he assured me that "it could not hurt my children unless it was baked in a cake and they ate the cake."

Our house had a forced heating and air conditioning system that was in constant use. It was February and all the windows were kept closed. The built-in storage area of my bedroom closet was directly above the heating system.

For the next two weeks, we slept in this bedroom while all of this "harmless" powder was in this closet. In the daytime, my 4-year-old son played in this room and I sewed.

Approximately 1 week later, I woke up at night clutching both hands over the area of my upper abdomen. I had sharp, stabbing pains in this area for several minutes, but soon went back to sleep and by morning had forgotten the incident.

Two weeks later, I looked in this built-in storage area of my closet. It looked as if it had snowed in there. All of my clothes were in this closet and I noticed that my black shoes were covered with a white dust. This closet was above a stairwell and the entire stairwell was also covered with this powder.

I decided to vacuum this powder out of the closet. After vacuuming for about five minutes, I developed blurred vision, violent stomach cramps, nausea, and just doubled over. I phoned the pest control company and was told by the secretary not to touch the powder, that a man would be sent to vacuum it up immediately, and that I wouldn't have to worry about it anymore. She also stated that he shouldn't have thrown this powder inside a house.

The same pest control operator came back and vacuumed the powder out of the closet. However, he was quite angry and he said that, "you have made a fool out of me at the shop."

We went about our business, thinking that we had reached the end of this little episode. Actually, it was just the beginning of an unending nightmare. I lost my appetite and gradually lost 14 pounds. I became nervous and irritable and had difficulty controlling my emotions. I became jaundiced and developed blurred vision that became worse each time I entered the closet.

In the morning, my eyelids were hard to open because of a sticky discharge running from my eyes and also because the eyelids were extremely edematous. My eyes, my skin, and my intestinal tract burned continuously. My abdomen growled so loudly that it awakened me several times a night. My abdomen hurt all the time and the abdominal skin itched.

At night, I would wake up and jump out of bed trying desperately to get my breath. I felt as though I were strangling due to a strange lump in my throat. By now, I had lost my appetite completely, was nauseated constantly, and finally I began to vomit.

For the first time in my life I thought that I would die. I was even more anxious for the welfare of my family. They were beginning to develop the same symptoms.

In addition, my 4-year-old son gradually developed a severe limp. This was later diagnosed by an orthopedic surgeon as Legg Perthes' Disease, a disease caused by loss of calcium. He had to wear a leg brace for a year and a half. All of us began to have light colored stools and my son had white stools. He would cry at night and point to his upper abdomen and say that he hurt there.

All of this seemed impossible to believe. My family physician had assured me that he had never heard of a single case of **DDT** poisoning. He felt that it might be an allergy and that I should "go home and forget the whole thing." I tried to do as he advised, but seeing my children and my husband with the same symptoms, I became more and more alarmed.

My own symptoms grew progressively worse. I noticed two fat chalasions near my eyes. The smaller one disappeared by itself, but the larger one had to be surgically removed. By now I had lost my sense of smell.

One night, the right side of my face felt anesthetized. I would wake up screaming with excruciating leg cramps and violent muscle twitching especially in the larger leg muscles. My arms and legs jerked at night while the inside of my head and spinal cord felt as if the nerves were ripping apart. My head jerked endlessly.

At this point, it was difficult to have a physician witness these violent symptoms because they seemed to reach their peak of violence at night when the body had been at rest. Insomnia is usually listed as a symptom of insecticide poisoning, but the reason for the insomnia was not explained.

Sleep seemed to be unobtainable. I was exhausted. I went from doctor to doctor hoping to find one who had heard of a similar case. I could not find medical help in San Diego. By now I was becoming hysterical not only because of my own nervousness and irritability, but also because I was worried about my family. What had I done to them? Where could I find help when no one would believe such a wild story as this? I now felt sure that our family suffered from severe insecticide poisoning even though some physicians had diagnosed me as a severe psychoneurotic.

I have two brother-in-laws. One owns a weed control company in Houston, Texas, and one of them is a chemist. We called them and they contacted the chief researcher of the Hazelton Chemical Company in Houston. He told us that we had definitely been poisoned and he advised us to immediately move out of that house and leave all of our belongings there since they were contaminated. We moved out.

At this point, I consulted with Dr. Francis M. Pottenger, Jr., of Monrovia, California, who had done research on pesticides as early as 1950. He was a specialist in internal medicine and metabolic diseases and had developed a special interest in insecticide poisoning. He was also at this time the air pollution chairman for the Los Angeles County Medical Society.

When I first consulted Dr. Pottenger in 1960, he said that he had put **DDT** in the ground ten years earlier and when he had dug it up he found that it still retained its original deadly properties. By 1960, Dr. Pottenger had a series of other patients with insecticide poisoning. He had established treatment programs and diagnostic tests that included fat biopsies.

Dr. Pottenger began my treatment that included dietary and vitamin therapy and injections of crude liver extract. At that time, Dr. Pottenger told me that a book was being written which would "rock the nation". *The Silent Spring,* by Rachel Carson, was published two years later. Dr. Pottenger had helped to write "Public Health Aspects of New Insecticides," which is one of Rachel Carson's references.

The Department of Agriculture sent a man down to examine our house after I filed a complaint with them. He said that he could do nothing since the **DDT** had been removed from the closet.

I heartily agreed with Mrs. Helen Nelson, State Consumer Counsel, whose primary recommendation was that the responsibility for protecting the public from pesticide pollution be placed on the Department of Public Health rather than on the Department of Agriculture. She also stated that the consumer is constantly exposed to pesticides in food, clothing, and even the air we breathe.

Dr. Pottenger arranged for a fat biopsy to be performed on me. The procedure was performed by a surgeon, Dr. Robert Wilson of Monrovia, California. The biopsy showed that I had 33 micrograms, or 33 parts per million of DDT. Dr. Pottenger stated that one part per million is equivalent to the weight of a 3 cent stamp.

We moved back into our house, thinking that we had decontaminated it. A year later, I had a second fat biopsy done by Dr. Robert Wilson. This one showed 45 micrograms or parts per million of **DDT**. We then threw away our furniture and for the second time we disposed of our mattresses and moved out of the house.

Two years later, in court, the pest control company admitted that this was a commercial concentration of 50 percent **DDT**. The manufacturer's directions stated that this powerful concentration should never be used in a house, but only in an attic or under a house. If one had to inhale the fumes, he was advised to go outdoors at least once every hour.

A year and a half later when we went to court, the defendant requested that I have a physical examination. During the next 8 days, I went through the usual tests given for a routine physical exam. I noticed that most of these tests were the same tests that I had written lab sheets for in 1945 when I was a student at Mercy Hospital.

It was clear to me that I was being examined by a team of doctors who had never heard of insecticide poisoning, except by ingestion, and whose tests certainly could not prove otherwise. Although the doctor was an allergy specialist he could not do an allergy test for **DDT** poisoning since he had never heard of one. How could he possibly diagnose something that he had never heard of nor believed existed? I feel that cases such as mine are happening every day and they are undiagnosed because of insufficient knowledge of pesticide poisoning by the medical profession.

For example, Billy Casper, an American professional golfer, was diagnosed with allergies when he played on golf courses. How can anyone diagnose Billy Casper's condition as an allergy when there was not an existing allergy test for pesticides? If he had a fat biopsy done and it proved that his body fat harbored pesticides, then a diagnosis of pesticide poisoning could be valid.

He played golf on the best golf courses where pesticides were undoubtedly used in large quantities. Billy Casper could determine for himself which courses were heavily sprayed and he tried to avoid those golf courses. It is for this reason that he omitted playing on the golf courses in Florida on his tours.

Since the allergist examining me, by his own admission, had never heard of a case of pesticide poisoning, except by ingestion, he and his chief psychiatrist felt I was psychoneurotic. So with this diagnosis we did not stand much of a chance to win our case in court.

However, I felt that it had now become a moral issue. If I could make others aware of what was really happening, I might save the lives of others. As my lawyers explained to me, this was a medical battle and even they had not heard of such a case. Each juror was asked if he had ever had any adverse effects from insecticides before he could qualify as a juror. Even the judge said, as the lawyers approached the bench, "In view of her condition....." He was referring to my mental condition as he had heard the psychiatrist describe it.

Much has been discovered about pesticides since this trial in March 1962, which leads us to question the effects of pesticides on man. As time goes by, it is my opinion pesticides will gradually contaminate our environment and all living things will unknowingly be affected.

The man who told me about Dr. Pottenger's work on pesticides was an ex-navigator for the Air Transport Command during World War II. Each time his plane landed, the crew was kept in the plane with a **DDT** mist for 15 minutes to delouse them.

Now, 20 years later, he still becomes ill every time he is exposed to pesticides. The pesticides cause him to have excruciating joint pains and the other symptoms associated with **DDT** poisoning, especially the feeling of strangling at night. Each repeated exposure brings about reoccurrence of the symptoms of pesticide poisoning as the body seems to go through a definite cycle as it tries to rid itself of the poison. I find that this is true in my own case.

On March 24, 1966, the San Diego Chapter of the American Society of Safety Engineers held a symposium at the Islandia Hotel in San Diego. One of their guest speakers on pesticides was the toxicologist who had testified against me during my lawsuit. He showed slides of the harmful effects of **DDT** poisoning which he swore didn't exist four short years before when he made a special trip from Los Angeles to testify against me.

I reminded him of his testimony against me in March of 1962 while he showed the slides of the now harmful effects of **DDT**, the same symptoms that I testified had affected us. I then suggested to him that he sleep with **DDT** in his bedroom closet and that he eat it as he had fed it to the prisoners and then, and only then, would he fully understand how treacherous it really was and still is! Needless to say, he was quite shocked and angry.

An experience such as this causes one to wonder what effect pesticides have on others, especially children. It has been scientifically established that even the penguins in the Antarctic, thousands of miles away from any actual spraying, have pesticides in their body fat. I cannot help but wonder how much the school children in this country have in their body fat after repeated "doses" from kindergarten through college and who have never eaten foods that were not sprayed.

Some of the greatest people I know in San Diego have contracted Alzheimer's disease. When I was a practicing nurse I never had a patient with Alzheimer's disease. I am devastated when I walk around my wonderful neighborhood and see my friends and neighbors with Alzheimer's. My best friend, Jean Neisewander, is blind because of macular degeneration. Was that brought on my pesticide poisoning?

I have asked the Harvard Medical Research team why the medical profession did not stop this insane poisoning of you and your children. Did the chemical companies buy off the medical profession or was it just the money made from the parade of patients coming into their examining rooms?

In my 70 years of experience as a nurse, I never heard of pesticides or flame retardant poisoning in our furniture and now in our food. Your generation has been fooled! Poison is poison as anyone knows and the pest control people who have no conscience know, but try to fool you.

When I sued a local pest control company in 1960, Dr. Frances Pottenger, who assisted Rachel Carson when she wrote *The Silent Spring*, told me "man will pollute himself out of existence" and that is exactly what is happening.

Today, out of the mouths of children we are hearing, "Stop the Poisoning of our food." Stop the chemical companies. Will these words be 60 years too late? The damage is done. My generation was fortunate to have organic food, unpolluted water and a beautiful earth, just as God made it!

Parents that I talk with today are horrified when they realize how they, and their children have been poisoned.

In 1960, when asked by my Attorney Sidney Stutz how I could get rid of the poisons the judge didn't believe the answer when Dr. Pottenger answered him, "by getting pregnant."

Dr. Pottenger told us then that if I had another baby, 95 percent of the poison would go to the baby and if I nursed the baby, 100 percent of the poison would transfer. Hearing this I was shocked. Therefore, I never had any more children. This is why I know that the multi-generational poisoning of you and your children is systematically destroying our world.

I am now 91 years old. You would be amazed if you knew how much poison could already be stored in your body. Ask Dr. Nan Kathryn Fuchs and all the young pediatricians. They know what I have said for years is the truth. I am writing you now so you have the answer for all generations that come after I am gone.

I happen to have been part of the original Nurses' Health Study group for 38 years. As I said to the most quoted Harvard Nurses' Health Study, your researchers are too young to know what happened.

However, this 91-year-old guinea pig can tell you. This hasn't happened because of coincidence. When I was poisoned by **DDT** I made a commitment to God to tell you the truth.

Chapter Two
My Nursing Career

God could not be everywhere; so he created mothers. Thank you, God. Mothers are the greatest people on earth as far as this old OBGYN nurse of 70 years is concerned. Women are wonderful. As I told the male doctors when I was Head Nurse in Mercy Hospital's delivery room, "Don't be too big for your britches. Just remember, you wouldn't be here without women. We old nurses have paid our dues a dozen times over and have gotten very little credit for our work." This book is also for you nurses.

Three years ago, the Nurses' Health Study wrote in large red letters on an envelope addressed to me, "We need you." At first I thought that it was a joke because I was then 88 years young. I wrote a 27-page letter back to them telling them what it was like in my world.

I said, "Who am I to tell the Nurses' Health Study anything?" Then I realized that those people doing the research are probably too young to know anything except what they learn on the computer.

In my letter I said, "The problem between you and me is the generation gap." The AARP Bulletin published their version of the generation gap.

In the report, Tom Brokaw was quoted as saying, "My generation was the greatest generation society ever produced." Now when I mention an ache or a pain I am being told by doctors, "You're getting old, you just have to live with it." Maybe yes and maybe no!

As Sarah Edelston Hiner, President at Bottom Line Publications, puts it, "Every time a doctor utters these words I hit the roof. There's no such thing as...nothing we can do...."

We worked darn hard during our lives. Don't we deserve a LITTLE bit of respect when we reach a certain age, dear friend? You bet we do! Sarah is very young and beautiful like you ladies in the Nurses' Health Study and you deserve the truth!

In my August 10, 2012, letter to Susan Hankinson R.N., I wrote, "I laughed when I read, 'We need you' on your envelope. I am no longer laughing because I realize that my 70 years as a nurse are very important. I can fill the generation gap! We need to look back and ask what happened in the nursing profession from January 8, 1945, until August 2012. In my opinion, they loused up the nursing profession, that's what happened!"

When I wanted to further my nursing career in my early career, I approached San Diego State College. I was informed that I could not enter their nursing program even though I had years of nursing experience in San Diego, California, as Head Nurse in Mercy Hospital's delivery room. San Diego State University couldn't let me earn a B.S. degree because they already had six nurses in their nursing program and they didn't want any more nurses. Can you believe that! I was 46 years old at that time.

When I became Head Nurse at Mercy Hospital in 1948, I had only worked for 6 months in the delivery room as a student nurse. The war had ended and America was getting back on its feet.

At that time, Mercy Hospital was delivering 500 babies a month. America was getting back on its feet and the baby boom was a direct result of it. As Head Nurse, I earned 195 dollars a month even though I worked countless hours.

When I married my husband, Walter Fiedler, he had a little one bedroom house in Coronado, San Diego, California. I worked the 3:00 p.m. to 11:00 p.m. shift. We were so busy that it was closer to midnight when I finally finished my day.

At the end of the day, I happily got in my 1937 Dodge with a rumble seat and rode down to catch the ferry to go back to Coronado, Island. This car was so old that the doors didn't lock and it had no heater.

When I arrived on Coronado I would drive down Orange Avenue to my street. The only street that had a white line was Orange Avenue. When I turned off Orange Avenue all the other streets were black top. If you have ever seen the fog in Coronado at 1 o'clock in the morning you would understand my dilemma. I actually couldn't find my house way down on G Street.

One night, I turned too soon and I ended up in a driveway of the fire station in spite of all its bright lights. Ironically, my husband, a building contractor, built the fire station that is still there.

We had very little money because he was in the Navy. He was stationed on the U.S.S. Bismarck Sea that was bombed by the Japanese. There were 800 men on that ship stationed off Iwo Jima and only three hundred men survived.

Walter was on the top deck and he had to jump in the water or die. Fortunately, he was an expert swimmer and so he survived. After the men abandoned ship the Japanese planes kept coming back and shooting the men that were trying to survive in the rough waters. My husband said the experience was hell.

A sailor on another ship took a picture of the U.S.S. Bismarck Sea when it was on fire and he gave Walt that picture which I still have.

When World War II was over, the men got out of the military about the same time. There were not many jobs so my husband bought a Monterey fishing boat and put an automatic pilot on it. He was fishing by himself for weeks at a time. I went back and forth by myself from Coronado to Mercy Hospital, often returning home at 1 o'clock in the morning. This is why Sarah Edelston Hiner, President of Bottom Line Publications, says, "We have paid our dues a dozen times over." I would say hundreds of times over.

I play Bridge at MCRD, a military base in San Diego, with the oldies-but-goodies like me, 91 years and older. We have such fun! Three of these wonderful ladies were Rosie-the-Riveter, like I was, and Brandy Costello was a Cadet Nurse like I was. We laugh at this generation that whine if they don't have five or six red Cadillacs, a fancy house, and a husband to help them. Not we old nurses!

Many of Mercy Hospitals' nurses were called "old maids", but I call them angels. They worked very hard and had very little money, no health insurance and no retirement pay. Nothing! Many nurses worked under brutal circumstances. However, they didn't complain. They were wonderful to all the patients and taught their student nurses with love and compassion.

I was on night duty with an older, gray-haired nurse, Miss McGovern, the sweetest little lady, taking care of about fifty patients. Miss McGovern's dream was to have a shelf full of purses. Some chance on her salary!

Mercy was a 500-patient hospital and at that time the only treatment they knew was bed-rest. At three o'clock one morning, I smelled smoke. I had an image of the hospital catching on fire, but I didn't want to frighten my head nurse, the elderly Miss McGovern.

We had two compress units on this floor and I thought that one of them might have a short circuit. I ran down the hall and found the first one was okay. I was running to find the other compress unit when I looked in a patient's room and saw that the patient in the room had been smoking a cigar and when he fell asleep the cigar caught his mattress on fire! There was no 911 and no time to call for help. The patient was a Mexican man that weighed about 200 pounds and was in a full plaster of Paris cast. He was asleep and he spoke no English.

What was a terrified nurse to do? I grabbed a pillow and put out the fire, what else? This man was now awake and sweat was rolling off his face. After I put out the fire, he motioned for me to bend down, and he kissed me and whispered, "Gratias." He spoke no English and I spoke no Spanish, but a kiss or a hug is all a nurse could expect!

The next morning, I told Sister what happened. She said to write an incident report. I didn't see myself on television telling every one of my good deed--Probably because there were no televisions at that time.

Where would you get more of an education than in a hospital? Well, I guess better than a college where they don't need more than six nurses in their nursing program.

Then the academics world came up with another debilitating decision. Nurses could no longer work as RN's unless they had a B.S. degree. These educators did not understand the importance of practical experience and one-on-one care. They failed to see this important aspect.

Well, this decision crippled the nursing profession. It limited the skill sets by placing purely academically educated nurses in the care role that requires practical experience. Today, I walk through a hospital and see nurses at the computers and not much hands-on-nursing that the patients loved and required to get well.

Every nurse was terrified enough at first in surgery. One time the Head Nurse sent us down for lunch. We had to walk through minor surgery in order to leave the surgical area. Well, the surgery door flew open and the Chief of Surgery yelled, "Nurse!" Since we all knew that he was "a god" and he had his personal scrub nurse. So I said, "I'll call her."

He pointed his sterile gloved hand in my face and said, "I mean you!" No one had ever heard the words, "sexual harassment." So he stood behind me and screamed at me telling me how I must scrub. Then in his gruff manner informed me that we were going to do a phrenectomy.

My classmate and I had never heard of such a thing, but into surgery we went. He blasted out orders to us. My classmate was a 6-foot, skinny, terrified blonde. In the middle of the surgery, I looked at her and I said, "Mary Lou, are you all right?" She said, "No. I'm going to faint!" Somehow, we made it through the intimidation of our first surgery.

In 1946, when I was a student in my first OB rotation, women were not OB GYN doctors. All doctors were men and most nurses were women. When women gave birth, it was difficult for a male doctor to understand the needs of the expectant mother. These patients were terrified enough and I'm sure would have preferred a woman doctor.

When my daughter said she would like to be a nurse, I told her, "With all your brains you could be a doctor." She is 62 years old and a retired Obstetrician. Thank God for women doctors! After she graduated from the University of Southern California, where they had a 1,000 deliveries a month, she was certainly well qualified.

I retired from nursing to have my family, but went back to work in Mercy's delivery room after they were grown. I really hadn't planned on returning to work after retiring for 20 years. I was walking in Fashion Valley Shopping Center one day when I met two of my former students, Jean Vesey, who was now O.B. Supervisor, and Betty Wheeler, who was now Head Nurse in O.B. They said, "Jeri, why don't you come back to work?"

I replied, "You must be kidding, after 20 years?"

Jean said, "Jeri. You forgot more than these kids ever learned."

I took a serious look at what they had said. I was really bored sitting at home after my kids went off to college. So I took an RN refresher course. I told the instructor that I would like to take my 6 weeks clinical in the O.B. ward.

Mercy had built a new hospital and I had never been in it. I took the refresher course and did the 6-week clinical in Mercy's emergency room. What an experience that was! Every morning, I scrubbed in minor surgery and every afternoon I helped with the emergencies. I was doing okay until they brought in a beautiful baby that died of crib death. I could handle everything except the death of a child.

If you go into Mercy Hospital, you will see a beautiful stained glass window donated by the Nicholas family. It is in memory of Nicholas. This very prosperous heart-broken family donated the entire beautiful chapel in Mercy Hospital in gratitude to the Sisters of Mercy. God bless them all.

After I finished the refresher course, I volunteered to work at Mercy. However, they said that they would have to pay me because their insurance wouldn't cover me unless they put me on their payroll. I had volunteered at the Navy Hospital and was told the same thing. Many years ago, many women came into the hospitals and volunteered in many of the departments and they were greatly appreciated by the staff nurses.

The Sisters of Mercy were eventually put out of business because of insurance concerns. A new system of administration had taken over the hospital and set new protocols for medical care. A new mindset was established when men from foreign countries didn't want men doctors examining their wives. It was about that time women were entering the medical field to study as doctors.

Today there's hope for the nurses in California. Having been a nurse for 70 years, I have been in the trenches and I know the truth! The older nurses did not receive enough credit from the doctors for their dedication and hard work nor were they paid a decent salary. There were no benefits and the doctors had the last say so in everything.

I know it was the nurses who really had the hands on knowledge about their patients. They kept the patients and hospitals going. The doctors back then thought they were gods and bedside manners and teamwork did not exist. Doctors treated their nurses poorly.

Actually, I believe that this generation of women have outdone themselves! Can you imagine a woman mayor! One of San Diego's women mayors was my first delivery.

I was in the delivery room one day and all 14 beds were full of screaming women in labor. "When their hour had come" it was hell for these mothers. The Caucasian women said, "Oh my God." The Jewish women said, Aye, Aye." The black women said, "Lord have Mercy!" One Chinese woman kept jumping off the stretcher and would squat in the corner. I think she had the right idea. It would be easier to push if you were sitting up. And so life went on.

Today, we have women lawyers, doctors, politicians, newspaper reporters, a woman Chief of Police and all the wonderful women police officers, women in the IRS Department, women judges like Judge Judy.

Judge Judy recently appeared on the *Dr. Oz Show*. She told how she had divorced her husband, Jerry, and then remarried him. Her comment, "Men!" said it all.

The man's world I knew was a stinking world. Women had no say, but now they run the show and well they should! Why not, they're brilliant, beautiful, and intelligent, and many men are jealous of them. Can you imagine Mary Barra as the first female chief executive officer of General Motors, and Michelle Howard first black 4-star Admiral?

Mia Angelo said, "There are none so blind as those who shall not see." Dr. Martin Luther King had a dream and so did his wife Coretta. Oprah Winfrey's beautiful farewell speech said it all. She spoke not only for black women, but also for all women and children that have been abused. She also said there is a God and she spelled it GOD. The Clippers made money for their boss, but were disgusted with his racist remarks. However, a judge ruled that his wife could sell the team. Hooray for women!

Sixty Minutes had a wonderful program on the 90-plus-year-old people. Finally, they are realizing, as Tom Brokaw said, "We are the best society ever produced." I am the luckiest woman alive to be in that wonderful generation.

Sean Hannity at Fox News asked, "What ever happened to decency? Too many of my generation died and the 'me' generation took charge." So sad!

As Dr. Richard Riley said, "They forgot to teach this generation morals."

I told the nurses in my letter to the *Nurses' Health Study* that George Bush Senior and his wife Barbara are my heroes. I have since seen his "Family Album." These are my kind of people! They raised a wonderful family. They are givers. They can never give enough of themselves.

At George Bush's birthday party the actor Chuck Norris asked, "How do you measure success?"

I would say to answer that, the wonderful families like the Bush family, Ronald Regan's family, Mitt Romney's family. What a beautiful family that is. I was fortunate to meet Mrs. Romney at the La Jolla Country Club at a Christmas party. She is more beautiful in person than on television. What a mother! She ignores her own illness and worries about every other family.

My patients were the best just like the women of the O'Connor family. One of these women came in the hospital just about every year and were thrilled to have a healthy child, a gift of God.

Then there was the Considine family. Mrs. Considine told me that I was her nurse. She had eleven children, eight of them born at Mercy Hospital. My daughter delivered their grandchildren. People-helping-people. What a privilege to know such fine people.

Let's hear it for nurses. Dr. Oz calls nurses the unsung heroes of the medical profession. They are always there when someone needs them. Johnson & Johnson has a television commercial showing a nurse running to help a man who was injured in a motorcycle accident.

Another commercial shows a male nurse singing to a little girl with a kerchief on her head meaning that she lost her hair because of cancer treatment. I could not work in pediatrics again after I had my own children. I still see the beautiful black 10-year-old girl that died in my arms when I was in pediatrics in 1947.

I feel the pain when I see John Walsh on television. The loss of his son ruined his life and I can see the sadness in his eyes and it breaks my heart. How can any monster kill an innocent child?

Dr. Keith Ablow, Chief Psychiatrist for ABC News said in disgust after the Newtown massacre, "Psychiatry stinks!" So does our injustice system that can't protect our children!

In 1960, my supervisor, Sister Mary Adrian, said, "This country doesn't take care of its own." Sister Mary was from England. That's putting it mildly. This "me" generation doesn't give a damn about anyone but themselves. The nuns were against abortions because they knew that all God's children have a right to life.

What a difference in people, this "me" generation is. I went to play Bridge to fill in for a friend that was ill. I sat down at the Bridge table and a loud-mouth woman started in telling us that she had a right to choose! I told her she had a right to go to hell and surely will!

The other person at the Bridge table was a lovely lady named Nan. I had never met her before and she told me that she had worked with Dr. Timothy Riley. Dr. Riley was an intern at Mercy when I was working there.

After I left, I heard that he became very ill, but thank God he survived. He delivered my granddaughter, Kelly. Another wonderful doctor! Dr. Michael Egan was an intern and he delivered my granddaughter, Brooke.

Many doctors are finally speaking out about the hazards of chemicals and pesticides and what they are doing to us. What fantastic people they are! It's past time that they receive praise for doing God's work and the nurses deserve praise as well. These are the givers. What would society do without them? They work so hard to become professionals and now because of National Health Care System Obama Care, the medical profession is fouled up, and the doctors and nurses are giving up. These doctors and nurses are disgusted with medicine as it is today.

On the other hand, as Dr. David Samadi says, "There are 185,000 medical mistakes a year." Dr. Oz tells us not to go to hospitals. One doctor calls this generation of medical care, "the cut, poison and burn care!" In my generation, hospitals were the places to go and you could expect excellent care. Not anymore!

Now many of the newer doctors are listening to what Hippocrates said, "Let food be thy medicine and let medicine be they food." My mother could have told them that. We are Italian.

The conclusion of many in the medical profession nowadays is just what Hippocrates told us, and what my mother taught us. She went all the way through the fourth grade, but she taught me the Mediterranean diet. Isn't that the conclusion of the Nurses' Health Study and every other study?

My mother had one book, "You are what you eat" by Dr. Frederick Stare and she cooked by his directions. That's why I am so healthy at 91 years of age and so are my other 90-plus-year-old friends. We grew our own foods and cooked and exercised, or more commonly known, we worked for a living. We did our own housework and I still do. I even do windows.

When I was about 5 years old, we had a restaurant and a gas station in Brookhaven, Long Island, New York. My mother and I cooked everything from scratch. I went across the street and picked organic, unpolluted blueberries and we made and froze blueberry pies. I climbed the apple trees and we made and froze apple pies. We sold a slice of pie for 10 cents. I went down to the bay and dug clams and we made clam chowder. All food was natural just as God made it and we loved doing it. We had so much fun. The doctors, especially the Italian doctors, know all about how important diet is just as my mother did. The Italian doctors learned this from their Italian mothers.

Dr. Nicholas Perricone made his fortune teaching the correct way to eat. Dr. Victor Marchione, "The Food Doctor" tells you what my mother taught me. Dr. Steven Sinatra, a world famous cardiologist gave up his practice and wrote the *Kitchen Confidential* cookbook. Dr. Joel Fuhrman's book *Eat to Live* is a national best seller. Dr. Oz was Dr. Fuhrman's classmate in medical school and wrote in Dr, Fuhrman's book *Eat to Live, A Medical Break-through.*

There is no question in my mind that it will work for you. I love Dr. Fuhrman who dedicated his book "To my mother, Isabel, for all her love and sacrifice and my father, Seymour, for instilling in me an interest in superior nutrition." The truest statement of all is in the Forward of *Eat to Live* written by his classmate, Dr. Mehmet Oz:

"Although the United States is the most powerful nation on earth, the one area in which this country does not excel is health and the future is not bright. Almost a third of our young children are obese, and many do not exercise. No matter how much information becomes available about dangers of a sedentary lifestyle and a diet heavily dependent on processed foods, we don't change our ways. Americans should be able to translate financial wellbeing into habits that lead to longer and better lives, untroubled by expensive and chronic medical illness. Yet in the United States, as well as Western Europe, Russia and many other countries, the majority of adults are overweight and undernourished. While high-quality nutrition is readily available throughout the United States, the American public, rich and poor, is drawn to eating unhealthy food. Indeed the list of top calorie sources for Americans include many items I do not consider "real foods", including milk, cola, margarine, white bread, sugar and pasteurized processed American cheese." 1

In another part of the Forward of *Eat to Live,*"Dr. Oz continues:

"With the publication of Dr. Joel Fuhrman's book, outlining a perfectly rational, straightforward and sustainable diet, I believe we are witnessing a medical breakthrough.

"I am a cardiovascular surgeon infatuated with the challenge and promise of "high tech" medicine and surgery. Nonetheless, I have become convinced that the most overlooked tool in our medical arsenal is harnessing the body's own ability to heal through nutritional excellence."[2]

This is the truth as I see it. We are going back to how I lived and how the Japanese, Chinese and many other societies live. Active lifestyle, unpolluted food, clean water, fresh air. That's why I am writing this book.

Dr. Oz has expert after expert on his show telling you how polluted everything has become. It's no surprise to me or to the holistic doctors! I was there 91 years ago in Brookhaven, Long Island, New York. It was a beautiful, clean, unpolluted area just as God intended it to be. My mother told me what to eat. She lived to be 95 as did her sister, Mary, who grew up in Hoboken, New Jersey. We didn't have to worry about how much pesticides we were eating since there were no pesticides. We didn't have to worry about flame-retardants all around us and in our food, BPA in our cans and Teflon in our cooking utensils.

Thank God for the holistic doctors like Dr. Mark Stengler. He is one of my doctors and he is the spokesman for Prevention Magazine. He agrees that our food is polluted. That's why he puts up his own supplements. Many doctors are doing that. I have a cupboard full of Dr. Mark Stengler's wonderful products.

Dr. Julius Whitaker is an M.D., but he saw all the problems with medicine today so he started his famous "Wellness Clinic." I also went to his wonderful clinic. He calls his patients and gives us his recorded messages. He also puts up his own supplements. These doctors are trying to supply unpolluted supplements since the food in this generation is far from the unpolluted food of my generation.

Thank God for the women doctors. They are the saints that are trying to save our children, grandchildren and great-grandchildren. One of the women doctors is doing a fantastic service to humanity. She is a holistic doctor who has this entire pollution mess figured out. If you want to get the truth, read Dr. Nan Kathryn Fuchs, PHD, Editor-in-Chief, *Women's Health Letter*. Dr. Fuchs saw the need to help women. Now she has published *The 456 Most Powerful Healing Secrets*.

In the Introduction she wrote in part:

"There's a tug-of-war going on and your health is at risk. Business interests are pulling on one end, and science is tugging at the other. I'd be amazed if you're not confused and frustrated. To tell you the truth, I've found that most doctors are as well. It takes time to sift through current information and separate the hype from the real deal. Who has the time to read through technical scientific studies? Who calls up researchers and doctors to better understand the validity of their conclusions? Well, I do. In fact, this is precisely what I've been doing for over 30 years as a nutritionist and health writer.

"Did you know that a common garden herb can often stop the hot flashes that accompany menopause? You may not need to take hormones at all if this is your primary menopausal complaint.

"Are you aware that an overlooked mineral deficiency could be responsible for both an under-active thyroid and breast cancer? Not only is there a way to test for this deficiency, it isn't expensive and you don't need a doctor's prescription to get it.

"What can you do when you can't get a yearly flu shot or it doesn't work? I found a supplement that has kept my patients and me free from colds, flu, bronchitis, and pneumonia for the past four years." [3]

Today, we see women helping girls and women. The Harvard Nurses' Study is the most comprehensive study ever done on women. I remember my daughter telling me years ago that we need this study because all the research has been done on men-even on male rats. They finally figured out that men and women have different needs and if they must use the dangerous, toxic medicines, women need different dosages than men.

Was it Dr. David Samadi that said, "We need to rewrite the medical books?" I look at my medical books of 1945 and laugh. Every patient was told the best treatment was bed rest. They kept the mothers in bed for 10 days after delivery and by that time (the bed pan days) they were too weak to stand by themselves. It took two nurses to help them stand.

I'm sorry to say that I lost three beautiful mothers when I got them out of bed after the two weeks of bed rest. All 3 died of an embolus, or a blood clot. What an unnecessary loss! They never even got to take their babies home. Well, the doctors just didn't know and this is how we learned.

Then during World War II the hospitals were bombed and the frightened patients ran out of the hospitals and they recovered from whatever their medical problem was. So that did it! The order came through to get the patients up immediately after a delivery or surgery. Who could afford a 2-week stay in a hospital anyway?

Dr. Nan Kathryn Fuchs published *The Nutrition Detective*. In Section I of her next book, *The 456 Most Powerful Healing Secrets,* Dr. Fuchs tells you what had happened between my generation and her generation. In previous generations if a patient had been diagnosed with diabetes, doctors told patients they needed insulin and they would need it for the rest of their lives. The nurses wrote up their diabetic diet.

In her book, Dr. Fuchs explains how you can reverse chronic illness. Dr. Joel Fuhrman tells you how to cure yourself of diabetes with proper nutrition. Dr. Fuchs further explains, "There are more therapies and diagnostic tools available to keep you healthy than ever before. Some are so powerful that they can reverse or reduce the severity of chronic illness.

Still, you are probably hearing about most of them here for the first time. Why is that? Quite simply, many of them are secrets that even your doctor doesn't know about. There are studies to back up their effectiveness. However, there are not as many independent studies as those funded by pharmaceutical companies and big suppliers of diagnostic tools.

I was poisoned in my home by **DDT** and as a result I suffered extreme reactions when exposed to pesticide use. In 1965, I went back to college to work towards my B.S. degree in nursing. But before long I had to give up that idea because the college was continually being sprayed with a liquid pesticide and each time they sprayed, I became ill.

One particular day when they sprayed, I left. When I returned to the campus two days later, they had sprayed the liquid pesticide that became a powder and it had blown into my classroom. The powder was on the floor and the instructor's footprints could be seen in this powder. I called this to the attention of the dean who merely had it swept up. She obviously didn't quite understand the seriousness of repeatedly exposing the students, future mothers and fathers, to these poisons.

Several of the married students were pregnant at the time. I can't help wondering about the possible metabolic disturbances their babies may have suffered as a result. A letter I received from the San Diego Unified School System was an attempt to justify their so-called "safe" spraying program.

I would like to remind you that all of us who graduated before 1945 went to schools that had never been sprayed. Can we say that these pesticides are safe when we read three pages of actual case histories from as eminent an authority as Dr. C. C. Hargraves of the Mayo Clinic?

For example, he tells of a 10-year-old boy who developed acute leukemia shortly after an entire "bug bomb" to fight bees was used in their enclosed garage. He continues with 3 pages of similar tragic cases. Dr. Irma West of the Los Angeles Health Department and Dr. Francis Pottenger concurred.

In *The Silent Spring*, Rachel Carson says, "Today more American school children die of cancer than from any other disease." With evidence pointing to the fact that chlorinated hydrocarbons, of which pesticides are one, are so dangerous to humans.

We continually ignore this evidence simply because we must not have a weed or a bug around our schools, even if the bug happens to be beneficial, as lady bugs are.

After 25 years of spraying, many bugs have built up resistance to the sprays and, therefore, require more toxic sprays than ever before to be destroyed. The evidence can no longer be ignored. These sprays are a dismal failure. 4

In 1963, I spoke at a P.T.A. meeting about these dangers, and I noticed one woman looked astonished. After the meeting, she said that her best friend had died rather suddenly and the only thing they found in the room was a bug bomb. Her death was attributed to dehydration although she had been in excellent health until this fatal incident.

In my opinion, this was a misdiagnosis, as usual, from a doctor that never heard of pesticide poisoning. A woman at that meeting went on to become the President of the P.T.A. at a local high school and she instituted a program that eliminated much of the spraying at this school.

Two years later, when my daughter attended that high school, I called the principal. She said that they now had "a bumper crop of lady bugs and all we intend to spray is one tree down in the canyon to kill the red spider." In 1969, the principal was transferred and with her went her decreased spraying program.

After she left, they resumed the usual spraying program. The school nurse was asked to call me before they sprayed so that I could take my children home. The last time she called me, they had already started spraying with **chlordane**.

According to Dr. Pottenger, **chlordane** is 5 times more toxic than **DDT** and dangerous to inhale and can be absorbed through the skin. Even though the school still reeked of **chlordane**, a school authority decided that they had to spray a second time that same month. I believe this was also with **chlordane**.

The third time the school nurse called me, she said that this time they would use a different spray. So that makes a total of 3 times that the high school was sprayed just in the month of May alone. Many of the children stated that it made them sick. The junior high school that my son attended was also sprayed three times during May, but I do not know what sprays were used.

In *The Silent Spring,* Rachel Carson explains why methoxychlor and Malathion are not as safe as the city schools have been led to believe them to be. 5

The alternative would be to try to undo the damage we have already done by spraying, which has upset the balance of nature. If spraying were stopped, the natural predators would take over as they have at my house that has never been sprayed in the 8 years we have lived here. Our yard is filled with lady bugs which seem to eat the aphids and; therefore, my plants are far healthier than those of the city schools.

Many of these school children could be adversely affected weeks and even months after the spraying is done and no one would link their illness to the pesticides because pesticides can cause a delayed reaction. These children have not had the diagnostic test done to determine whether or not they have pesticide poisoning because a fat biopsy requires surgery and most parents would not consent to this. Also, no one takes into consideration the medications that these children are taking.

Regarding the warning of the interaction of chemicals, Rachel Carson states in *The Silent Spring,* "The individual exposed to **DDT**, for example, is almost certain to be exposed to other liver-damaging hydrocarbons, which are so widely used as solvents, paint removers, degreasing agents, dry-cleaning fluids, and anesthetics." 6

What then can be a 'safe dose' of **DDT**? This is true of all pesticides, many of which are more toxic than **DDT**. Also repeated exposures may finally cause death. No one can say which exposure may cause death. Rachel Carson refers to sprays as, "The hiss of death."

In 1960, Dr. Pottenger predicted a tremendous rise in hepatitis and; unfortunately, his prediction came true. He also pointed out the increasing numbers of cases of multiple sclerosis. Could these diseases be traced to the nerve and liver poisons known as pesticides"? Rachel Carson certainly believed that they could be when she suggested in *The Silent Spring,* "that the relation between a soaring rate of liver disease and the prevalence of liver poisons in the environment is no coincidence." 7

Several thoughts have occurred to me as a result of my experience. I could not sleep for more than half an hour on the mattresses in our house that had been contaminated without having violent muscular twitching. When I learned that it was impossible to de-contaminate a mattress, I wondered how many other people must unknowingly be sleeping on contaminated mattresses.

I know that sprayed poisons are retained by mattresses. When I tried to reupholster a chair 5 years after it had been removed from our contaminated house, I became violently ill for the second time.

During my trial against the pest control company, the pest control company stated that many mattresses were impregnated with a 5 percent solution of **DDT** as protection against bedbugs.

On one occasion, I observed new mattresses being loaded on a truck at a warehouse. The sign on the door of the truck aroused my curiosity so I checked in the telephone directory and found that this company specialized in sterilizing mattresses. This meant that the mattresses were being filled with poisons, rather than being sterilized in an autoclave.

I decided to learn how mattresses were constructed. I found that many mattresses have a solid sheet of foam rubber on the top and another sheet of foam on the bottom. Many mattresses as well as many pillows are 100 percent foam rubber. Foam rubber is porous and known to absorb very readily. It is logical that pesticides that are repeatedly used in homes would accumulate in the mattresses and pillows.

For example, whenever a house is fumigated to rid it of termites, the tent enclosing the house is filled with poisonous gas. The homeowners are instructed to remove all articles containing foam rubber. When foam rubber is used as padding under carpeting and throughout the construction of furniture how can it be removed?

A woman told me that a neighbor's house was fumigated and they neglected to remove one foam rubber pillow. When they moved back into the house a boy slept on this pillow and died.

The fact that such an incident can occur made me wonder if this could directly or indirectly cause "crib deaths" since it has now been proven conclusively that pesticides caused thousands of bird deaths and are responsible for the "fish kills."

Even if a house has not been fumigated, there is much spraying done around the house, in the yard, and in the gardens.

I have read some woolen mills routinely mothproof all their wools as do all woolen yarn companies and all wool carpet companies.

I also read that many synthetic carpets are also mothproofed even though moths will not eat synthetics. Dry cleaners proudly post signs on their windows that say, "We mothproof everything we clean."

Much of our bedding is moth-proofed and many people who have been told that moth crystals are harmless hang them in their bedrooms along with roach cakes and pest strips.

Insecticide impregnated shelf paper keeps the dishes and foods well contaminated and we are told on television that bug bombs kill at a distance of 50 feet and behind walls.

However, they neglect to say that these poisons are also getting into our body fat as well as household furnishings.

According to the experts, these commercials also tell us that 10,000,000 pets wear flea collars that can kill fleas up to 90 days at a distance of 3 feet away. How many children are sleeping in the same room or even the same bed as a pet wearing one of those flea collars? And if these poisons can kill at such great distances, why are they put right alongside our groceries, many of which are wrapped in paper and cardboard, as are the insecticides themselves?

The pharmacology department of the University of Rochester cautioned about using naphthalene, a substance used in mothballs and moth-flakes, for storing clothing of infants and young children. The Rochester people state that while mothballs themselves were a hazard with children simply because they look like candy and might be eaten.

With babies the naphthalene may be absorbed through the skin, especially if baby oil has been used on the skin. It can be highly toxic to an infant. This means it is highly toxic to a child before it can even walk. Babies crawl on mothproofed carpeting and put their hands and toys that have been on this carpeting in their mouths.

Even hospital administrators are so totally unaware of these dangers that they have their carpeting mothproofed each time it is washed. I feel that these practices should be stopped and the amount of spraying around homes, schools, and hospitals should be minimal or discontinued entirely.

If these poisons are adversely affecting me, now that I am sensitized to them, they are most certainly affecting others.

When we look at the children of today, we find that their mothers have been on a diet of sprayed food since 1945. It has now been scientifically established, through fat biopsies, that these chlorinated hydrocarbons not only accumulate in the body fat of the mother, but they are transmitted from the mother to the baby during pregnancy.

Therefore, for the first time we have a generation of babies that have accumulated poisons from the moment of conception.

One has to wonder what genetic damage will result in future generations. We must understand that once these poisons are used there is no way to remove them. So we must ask how much do babies pick up from their environment. I picked up twelve more micrograms of **DDT** in one year in a supposedly de-contaminated house, and children are more susceptible than adults.

There is nothing in their environment that does not contain pesticides after 25 years of spraying. Milk, babies' chief food, is supposed to have zero tolerance to pesticides, but as Rachel Carson tells us in *The Silent Spring*, page 162, "In actual fact residues turn up whenever a check is made."

Pesticides: In The World Around Us published in the San Diego Union Tribune about me, March 19, 1979, addressed this very issue exactly twenty years after my family was poisoned.

Pesticides: In The World Around Us
San Diego Union Tribune
March 19, 1979

Geraldine Fiedler had to practically smuggle her new living-room furniture into California from Oregon.

That is because California upholstered furniture makes her nauseous and dizzy due to materials manufacturers use to comply with the state law that upholstered furniture meet flame-resistant standards.

It's a long story, and one that began in 1959 when Fiedler's house was contaminated with **DDT** *deposited in her closet by a San Diego pest control firm. It saturated her clothes and circulated throughout the house via the heating system.*

Fiedler, a nurse at Mercy Hospital, had violent reactions and, to a lesser extent, so did her husband and two young children.

It was just the beginning of an unending nightmare. I lost my appetite and gradually lost 14 pounds. I became nervous and irritable and had difficulty in controlling my emotions. I became jaundiced and developed blurred vision which became worse each time I entered the closet . . . My eyes, my skin and my intestinal tract burned continuously . . . At night I would wake up and jump out of bed trying desperately to get my breath. I felt as though I were strangling due to a strange lump in my throat. I was nauseated constantly and finally I began to vomit . . . . "

Because of that 1959 experience Fiedler was sensitized to **DDT**, *a chlorinated hydrocarbon, and related chemical compounds. When she is exposed to one of them, the symptoms recur -- the nausea, burning, muscular spasms and dizziness.*

Unfortunately, Fiedler has found out through continuous bouts with the symptoms that these chemicals are all around her. And they have changed her life.

She cannot go into restaurants that have been sprayed recently with pesticides. She cannot use many detergents, soaps, cleaning products like floor wax, paint materials or even hair spray.

She had to stop going to her children's PTA meetings when the schools were being sprayed with pesticides, and she kept her children home at those times.

Last year she had to cancel a trip to New Zealand because she found out the jets had to be sprayed. It cost her a $340 deposit. But buying furniture has been her biggest problem.

California law requires upholstered furniture to resist bursting into flame when subjected to a smoldering cigarette. Many flame retardants used are chlorinated hydrocarbons or close relatives and some of the flame-resistant synthetic materials, like foam polyurethane, trigger a recurrence of symptoms in Fiedler.

According to tests done shortly after the pesticide poisoning occurred, she had a residue of 45 parts per million of DDT in her fat. That level could be considerably higher now since the body fat tends to store the poison with additional exposures.

Dr. Frederick Kutz, an ecological monitor of pesticides for the U.S. Environmental Protection Agency (EPA) in Washington, D.C., said that today, when pesticides are so much more common than they were 20 years ago, people average about five parts per million of ***DDT*** *in their system.*

Dr. Kutz said some people have greater resistance to pesticides and their bodies can contain much higher levels without harmful side effects. For instance, the EPA has found through repeated testing that blacks retain twice as much ***DDT*** *in their fat as whites after equal exposure.*

While very little is known about pesticide poisoning today, far less was known when Fiedler was stricken. She went from doctor to doctor hoping to find someone who could help.

She recalls, "I could not find medical help in San Diego. I was becoming almost hysterical, not only because of my own nervousness and irritability (brought on by the chemical) but also because I was worried about my family. What had I done to them? Where could I find help when no one would believe such a wild story as this?"

Eventually she found a researcher with the Hazelton Chemical Company who confirmed that she had been poisoned and was referred to a Monrovia doctor familiar with pesticide exposure who put her family on a high-protein diet with vitamin supplements.

Even today it is difficult to find physicians schooled in insecticide chemical poisoning. Most doctors just don't know about it . . . It's a unique area that's just now being explored," said Dr. Kenneth Cohen, a San Diego industrial hygienist toxicologist who lectures and provides expert testimony on chemical poisoning.

It happens a lot more often than we might think. An EPA survey of general admission hospitals throughout the United States found that about 40,000 patients were treated for pesticide poisoning from 1971 to 1973. A similar survey is now being conducted for 1974-75.

The problem, Dr. Kutz explained, is that the chemicals are all around us. They now permeate our atmosphere and there is no way to avoid them completely.

Fiedler is doing her best. To get around having to buy furniture treated with a fire retardant, she decided to have an interior designer reupholster her old furniture with untreated material.

But as soon as the reupholstered furniture arrived, the flu-like symptoms began to recur with increasing severity as each day passed. A chemical laboratory test of the material identified a high concentration of pesticides apparently from warehouse spraying somewhere in the life of the material before it arrived in San Diego.

Back went the furniture and for a year Fiedler and her family lived in a practically furniture-bare living room. Meanwhile, she checked several furniture manufacturers in other states for "untreated" sofas. She found the Oregon source.

Since the manufacturer could not sell the furniture to her directly (it would have violated California standards), he sold it to her brother who lives in Oregon. Her brother, in turn, turned it over to her and she "moved" her furniture into this state. (It is legal to "move" non-flameproof upholstered furniture here.)

She was not so lucky in replacing an 18-year-old mattress. Three years ago she bought a new one without a second thought until about nine nights after the new bedding arrived when she felt she was strangling. It finally occurred to her to read the mattress tag.

Sure enough, it said that flame retardant had been added. She found out later that federal standards require all mattresses sold to meet the "smoldering cigarette test", that is, not burst into flame under the heat of a smoldering cigarette.

She is not alone in her dilemma. Lorraine Back, an interior designer with Walter Broderick & Associates, said she had a request from a San Diego woman last week for a custom-made mattress because the woman said she was allergic to a store-bought mattress.

"But we can't make anything for anybody that doesn't meet California and federal codes," Back said. She added that she sympathized with the woman because her own hands itch, turn red or peel when she handles certain treated fabrics.

Rudy Slate, a local drapery manufacturer, is so allergic to the fabrics that his doctor told him to give up his job. Instead, he air-conditioned his office and only occasionally goes into the drapery room. When he does, he wears a respirator.

Federal regulations do allow someone with an allergic reaction to a flame-resistant mattress to get a nonflammable one "by doctor's prescription" -- but finding one is next to impossible and having one custom made is expensive.

Fiedler has mattresses sent from Arizona and she is happy she can breathe again and her muscular spasms have subsided. She even makes all her own clothes so she can buy dress material that she knows will not bother her.

When the nurse was interviewed, she emphasized that she was not telling her story to make people feel sorry for her, but to alert them to the dangers of these chemicals so they can avoid excessive exposure.

She gets upset when she walks into the supermarket and finds dog flea collars, fly strips or roach cakes alongside food. And she worries about children attending schools that have been sprayed.

"They didn't spray schools when I was a young girl and look how much **DDT** *I've accumulated . . . Imagine how much our children will have in their systems by the time they grow up."*

She is worried that the combination of treated mattresses, federally mandated flame-proof children's bedclothes, sprayed schools and now the threat from the federal government that all upholstered furniture be flame-resistant is creating a poison time bomb for future generations.

Even though **DDT** *is banned from use now it is throughout the environment and studies have shown that a pregnant woman passes the poison on to her child at birth.*

Fiedler has contacted the Consumer Product Safety Commission both in opposition to its proposed new flammability standards for furniture and the use of polyurethane foam which releases a lethal gas when it burns.

But proponents of the measure point out that each year 3,200 people are injured and 800 die in upholstered furniture fires; more than half of the deaths are attributed to cigarettes. It appears unlikely the CPSC will back down from its proposal.

Meanwhile, there have been hopeful advances in the treatment of those persons with pesticide buildups in their body tissue. Treatment so far is experimental, but some methods, one involving chemotherapy, have withdrawn successfully some of these chemicals from body tissues Dr. Kutz said.

But research also indicates, according to Cohen, that even if this material is cleared from the body tissues, the main damage was already done when the initial overexposure took place and the body's sensitivity is likely to continue.

Cohen strongly urges that one way to avoid mishaps is for people to read instructions thoroughly and follow them.

I was alerting readers just as the woman physician did in *The Fumigation Chamber,* and the World War II pilot, Hal Hunt, did when he wrote *My Experience with Pesticides,* and his wife, Ardath did when she wrote "Protect Yourself from Chemical Poisons," and just as Billy Casper did in his newspaper article telling why he doesn't play golf in Florida! You'll read about them later in this book. **No one listened!**

Chapter Three
Our Neighborhood

My husband was working on a house in Bay Park. The house was owned by a lovely family. The dad was the Assistant Police Chief in San Diego. After he sprayed chlordane under his house he became very ill.

My lovely neighbors, Ruth and George Meadows didn't have any children of their own but they loved everyone else's children and all of us loved them. They had a well taken care of backyard and served potluck dinners there. All kinds of meetings and parties were held at their house.

George went wild with supposedly safe chlordane. Because of that I called him "**Chlordane** Meadows." He had been convinced by a chemical company that the chlordane wouldn't harm anyone. No one asked him how much chlordane he had inhaled or absorbed through his skin. George was a retired Navy officer and he worked for my husband. George died in my husband's office at 50 years of age.

George Meadows lived down-wind from Hal Hunt. Every time George sprayed **chlordane**, the wind would blow into Hal Hunt's yard and Hal became deathly ill as he tells in his article below.

My Experience with Insecticides

By H. C. Hunt

April 13, 1963

As a navigator in the U.S. Air Forces Air Transport Command, Ferrying Division, stationed at Long Beach, California, during the year 1944-1945, I ferried airplanes to both Pacific and European theaters. The round trip took from two weeks to a month. Each time that we landed in a different continent, different country, and sometimes even a different island a bug bomb was sprayed in the plane before the doors could be opened and we could disembark.

The navigators made their way back to Long Beach on their own after every ferrying trip, so I would sit in the sprayed airplanes for at least 10 minutes to a half hour for at least four times in the 2-week South Atlantic trip to England and return. In addition, the sleeping quarters were always sprayed in Brazil and Africa for mosquitoes before going to bed and the mess hall was usually sprayed, as well as the latrines. Usually local civilian personnel were in charge of the spray detail.

Remembering back after a couple of trips it got so that my eyes watered heavily and my nose filled up during and after the spray. I always breathed through my handkerchief during the spray period but it didn't help much.

Near the end of 1945 I returned to upstate New York for nine months and felt in good condition. I returned to the University of California at Los Angeles in the fall of 1946 and seemed to be in relatively good health.

In 1951, I started to build my own house in my spare time. The location was on a hill in which the prevailing wind was from the ocean. Every couple of months I would end up in bed with terrific aches in all of my muscles and especially in my joints. My eyes hurt in back of them, it seemed, and I had a sort of lumpy feeling in the lower part of my throat and upper chest. I would wake up during the night feeling I was choking even after the muscle and joint aches had gone.

Looking back now, I realize that after the outside of the house was completed and while I worked inside the house I didn't have the attacks.

In 1955 I started building a garage in back and after working one week-end on the garage roof, I had the same type of attack again My wife discovered that our neighbor who was up-wind from us had liberally sprinkled chlordane on her lawn that weekend to kill the lawn moths.

I apparently had inhaled enough of the ***chlordane*** *powder to trigger off an attack. Once we saw the connection, my attacks could usually be traced to exposure to insecticides.*

For example, after having another bout on a weekend, when I was no longer working outside, inquiries at my office showed that the janitor had sprayed insecticide around the floor on Thursday night, which meant that I had breathed it all day Friday.

This also tied in with another problem I had during that period in which I drove to Los Angeles about once a month. After driving in the traffic for about an hour and inhaling the fumes my eyes and head would hurt so much that I would not be able to do the driving home to San Diego.

-S-
H. C. Hunt,
San Diego, California

This is important because Hal and Ardath Hunt knew Dr. Pottenger, and Ardath was my best friend. She was much more of an expert writer. We worked on this together for years. When Hal tells you that he became ill, that was when George Meadows, (I called him "**Chloradane**" Meadows) sprayed downwind it made Hal sick! They were close neighbors!

Ardath Hunt is Hal Hunt's wife and here is her article. Ardath and I wrote to Senator Waxman, CBS News when Dan Rather was anchor. Ardath was a writer and had several articles published. Hal died of Alzheimer's disease and Ardath died of heart disease. I can't do much without them or Dr. Francis Pottenger or Dr. Purvis Martin.

I am told **Chlordane** is probably the most commonly used control in buildings of all available insecticides. It is routinely used even in hospitals and is an extremely dangerous nerve and liver poison.

One wonders what could cause spasms in a baby that appears perfectly healthy. As I remarked earlier, the most frightening symptom I had was the feeling of strangling during the night and my children also complained of this symptom.

Yet none of the many doctors could see these spasms since they occurred only at night or when the body was at rest. How then could unsuspecting mothers see them in their babies when a physician could not detect them in a patient who has 45 micrograms as I have? It should be noted that "crib deaths" occur only at night or during naps--or in other words when the body is at rest.

When we check our other references we find that all other patients with insecticide poisoning complained of a "lump" in the throat or a constriction in the throat. Billy Casper speaks about his "throat tightening." All these patients complain about a "persistent sore throat, often followed by a persistent or recurrent feeling of constriction or a lump in the throat".

In an article, we find that the insecticide **endosulfan** caused paralysis of the breathing organs and suffocation of millions of fish in the Rhine.

In his deposition for my trial, Dr. Pottenger said this lump in the throat is an important symptom of pesticide poisoning and he calls it a "globus phenomena." If this can happen to an adult, why is it not worth considering in "crib deaths?"

What I am suggesting is that even though babies may not be getting a lethal dose of insecticides, per se, they could be getting enough to produce symptoms of edema such as Dr. Bergman mentions in his article, thus bringing about the spasm of the larynx.

As more is discovered about pesticides, more questions arise. For example, it has recently been discovered that the peregrine falcon and the California brown pelican face extinction because pesticides have removed too much calcium from their eggshells. This results in dangerously thin-shelled eggs that crush easily. If the removal of calcium in birds proves so disastrous, what effect does it have on humans?

My son had been in our house that was contaminated with **DDT** for approximately 2 months when he developed a severe limp that was diagnosed as Legg Perthes Disease. Dr. Morton Biskind states, "Several young children exposed to DDT developed a limp lasting from 2 to 3 days to a week or more."

All patients with insecticide poisoning complain of excruciating leg cramps. These leg cramps seemed similar to those I had experienced during pregnancy but were much more violent. The leg cramp I experienced during pregnancy were relieved by double doses of calcium. We were unable to relieve the leg cramps caused by the poisoning and each subsequent exposure to pesticides causes a repetition of this symptom.

Even today, my neighbors remember the horror we experienced. My dear friend Linda wrote me a letter February 10, 2015 to express her gratitude for my efforts on behalf of so many.

Dear Geri,

*You asked me a couple of questions starting with the Pest Control. Do I ever remember! Every time I saw a white truck with a running cartoon mouse on it, my brain did a mantra, "**DDT, DDT**..."*

My childhood was influenced by your passion, research and guts. The physical evidence and mental "ahahs" dovetailed with your constant updates to my parents. I listened to you. ...

*And I remember the moves you made. One you didn't mention was (if I've got this right a rented house) in a rather new neighborhood next to a canyon, Sierra Mesa maybe" Jeanie and I went for a walk. There was a squashed rabbit on the street. I remember because the neighborhood was like ours – yet foreign – and the dead rabbit added to my fear of familiar faces in unfamiliar places ... all a result of **DDT**. ...*

What I didn't realize was the extent of your pain. If I didn't know how it was, I assume the reasons are 2-fold. One that at my age I couldn't imagine such suffering and two (most likely) you soft pedaled the most horrible symptom around us kids. ...

You know, our house on Dorcas was built on an anthill that could not be vanquished. ... "The ants, the ants, the damned ants", my mother would say years later, having lived with the buggers for so long, but she never used anything stronger than vinegar on them. I don't think she was concerned about ant spray as much as she worried about its effect on your compromised system ....

-S-
Love Linda
P.S. You're one of the nurses" In the studies – famous work – I'm so proud of you.

Chapter Four
Protecting Yourself From Poisoning

Having worked in the nursing field and understanding the repercussions of exposure to toxins, I found myself and my family and friends placed in great danger. I was exposed to **DDT** and suffered from **DDT** poisoning that almost killed me.

I was unaware of what the effects of a pesticide would do to the human body until I suffered the symptoms of exposure and had to live through the treatment.

Whenever they sprayed at the public schools in the 60s' and 70s', I took my kids out of school but felt like a criminal to know the rest of the kids were being repeatedly poisoned. I went to the Education Center 5 times and they laughed at me. I was dubbed "The Spray Lady" and was certainly given no respect even though I was a nurse.

Every time they sprayed the schools with one poison or another some of the mothers would come to me and say that their children would become sick with flu-like symptoms.

Have you ever heard of misdiagnosis? After enough complaining about our kids being poisoned when the chemical companies would do nothing to stop it, I decided that whenever I saw them spraying this wonderful "non-poisonous" poison on your kids, I would slam on my brakes and go in and talk to the principal.

I went in and talked to a new principal at Bay Park school and she looked shocked and she went out and told the gardener never to spray the school again. So for the six years that my already poisoned son, Bill, was there they did not spray and everything was just fine as the schools were in my generation. They didn't need to be sprayed.

The new principal said she had just read an article in the New Yorker Magazine telling how unsafe these insecticides were.

My daughter attended Marston Jr. High School. I had already told them to call me before they sprayed so I could take her home. Jeannie hated for me to take her out of school since she was a straight "A" student and didn't want to miss any classes.

However, she didn't need to be poisoned just to be a straight "A" student--that is except for one "B+". One morning, I took Jeannie to an early morning class and the maintenance personnel were spraying two water trucks full of poison over the entire school. I asked one of the men what they were spraying and he said Chlordane. You can guess what I did next.

In the 1950's, schools were sprayed repeatedly with pesticides exposing the children and educators to high risks of toxins. When I discovered this practice and saw first-hand the effect, I fought to have the practice eliminated.

Whoever shouts the loudest gets heard! Giant corporations shout loudly with their advertising dollars. Finally, there are doctors of this generation who are saying exactly what Dr. Fuchs said. A major problem arose when chemical and pesticides were being utilized incorrectly due to lack of the understanding of their long reaching effects. The use of the chemical and pesticides has a useful function, but they are placing our children and ourselves at risk. Proposition 65 allows people to sell products that cause cancer and birth defects as long as this warning is placed on the product. That still does not protect the innocent by-stander who is exposed to toxic chemicals.

Nobody gave a damn what it did to you kids. Just so the chemical companies make more billions at our expense. Well, who do they think they're fooling? Not me! Dr. Oz is shocked to find so many pesticides and flame retardants in our food. I'm not. Didn't I tell you so in 1959? Remember me? I'm the "Spray Lady," as I was called by the San Diego school system.

In January 4, 1988 Berton Roueche wrote *Annals of Medicine,* an article about a woman physician. I loved her statement when she said her doctor treated her like a "brainless woman." Typical way women were treated in my generation.

October 10, 1967
Miss Geraldine Fiedler, R.N.
1512 Dorcas Street
San Diego, California 92110

Dear Miss Fiedler:

We felt that your letter voicing concern over spraying practices at the city schools deserved immediate investigation, rather than waiting for publication of a letter to call attention to possible harmful methods.

A spokesman for the school district provided the following information:

The school district for years has contracted with a professional extermination firm to inspect and do required services in school cafeterias once a year spraying in junior and senior high school home economics rooms.

"The contract also calls for the firm to perform service "as required." For example, if a swarm of bees alights on school grounds, a truck is supposed to rush to the scene and exterminate them. Ant infestations also develop around schools and getting rid of them is another example of the contract stipulations.

"With such exceptions as bee swarms, all spraying is done at times when students are not in school. Usually it takes place immediately after the school day, with rooms shut up during the night. Gardeners and custodians also perform certain spraying functions and these, too, are conducted at non-school hours.

"All procedures affecting health and food handling are done with the approval of the Health Department, which sends out its personnel to provide in-service training to school personnel. The school district's health education specialist, Dr. Gage Wetherill, prescribes what types of pesticides can be used at schools and school grounds and the use of arsenic is forbidden."

This would seem to eliminate any anxiety on the subject. If you can provide specific instances when spraying was done in the presence of children, however, we will be glad to pursue this further.

-S-
San Diego Unified School District
Education Center
Park and El Cajon Boulevards
San Diego, California 92103

May 14, 1969

Geraldine Fiedler, R.N.
1512 Dorcas Street
San Diego, California 92110

Dear Miss Fiedler:

Thank you very much for sending me all the clippings and articles on pesticides and other chemicals used for spraying. I am returning them to you as you requested.

I checked into the use of pesticides by the City Schools and found the following information in which I thought you might be interested.

The school district has always been concerned about the methods and timing of applications of both insecticides and herbicides as well as their toxicity. The use is far more important than the actual toxicity, and all reasonable precautions are taken to avoid contamination. There has been some correspondence with Dr. J. B. Askew, Director of Public Health, and the district has received his evaluation of the materials being used.

The material sprayed inside of buildings for the control of ants is ***Methoxychlor*** *in an oil carrier, one of the least noxious of toxic materials that can be used. It may even be sprayed in the air in food handling plants. Materials are rated by an LD (Lethal Dose) number. The number can be translated into the number of ounces of a 5% solution required to be consumed orally by a 50 pound child to cause ill effects. The LD 50 number for* ***Methoxychlor*** *is 6000.*

This means a lethal dose would require drinking 104 ounces, 3 quarts. The commonest material used on plants outside is ***Malathion****. It has an LD 50 number 2000. Of the materials listed for Dr. Askew, the lowest LD number, that is the most toxic, was* ***chlordane****. Its number was 350.*

This means it would require 6.6 ounces taken orally to cause ill effects. However, and unfortunately, there is no way to gauge the amount of insecticide necessary to make one sick or nauseated, particularly since individuals are so variable in their susceptibility.

As a result of Dr. Askew's recommendations, for several years now we have used no arsenical snail bait, and we no longer use ***lindane*** *or* ***toxaphene*** *because they are highly volatile and their fumes are more apt to cause a feeling of sickness than most other compounds.*

In addition, the gardeners have been instructed not to do their spraying while the children are around in order to minimize airborne odors which may bother highly sensitive persons.

If you have any further questions, please call me. Thank you for your continued interest in the schools.

-S-

At least they didn't fog San Diego with poison like they did in Texas and many of the other states. When I told my beautiful friend Mona McMinn, how I tried to stop them from spraying the kids in school, she said that's what happened to her in Texas when she was in school.

When my sister-in-law, Norma, and I were in Little Rock, Arkansas, we got up at 5:00 a.m. to catch a plane and they fogged the city and we were exposed.

For many years the parents would come to me and tell me that when the schools were sprayed and the kids were exposed and became sick, the problem was misdiagnosed as the flu instead of poisoning.

If they hadn't shut women up, you wouldn't have pesticides in your food as well as flame retardants, mercury in your fish, arsenic in your apple juice, lead in paint and in gasoline, hormones in your milk, **PBA** in cans, and now radiation in fish.

As Dr. Fuchs asks, "Do we need to say goodbye to one of our most healthful foods fish?" Dr. Fuchs is a holistic doctor and she has been telling women for 30 years what is happening. I have been trying for 70 years! She couldn't get through to the greedy chemical companies either!

Chapter Five
Pesticides

History of Pesticide Use

The practice of agriculture began over 10,000 years ago in Mesopotamia which is part of modern day Iraq, Turkey, Syria and Jordan where edible seeds were gathered by the population. [8] Cultivation of wheat, barley, peas, lentils, chickpeas, bitter vetch and flax soon developed. In China, rice and millet were domesticated whilst about 7500 years ago rice and sorghum were farmed in the Sahel region of Africa. [9] The need to avoid famine due to disease and pests was a grave concern to ancient farmers.

The first recorded use of insecticides is about 4500 years ago by Sumerians. They used Sulphur compounds to control insects and mites. The Chinese about 3200 years ago used mercury and arsenical compounds for controlling body lice. [10] Smoke was also used to control pests. [11]

Up until the 1940's inorganic substances such as sodium chlorate and sulphuric acid or organic chemicals derived from natural sources were widely used in pest control. [12]

The growth in synthetic pesticides accelerated with the discovery of the effects of DDT, BHC, Aldrin, diekdrin, endrin, chlordane, parathion, captan and 2,4-D. DDT was used widely and appeared to have low toxicity and reduced insect-borne diseases like malaria, yellow fever and typhus. 13

In 1946, it was reported that house flies had developed a resistance to **DDT**. In 1949, Dr. Paul Muller won the Nobel Prize in medicine for discovering insecticidal properties harm to non-target plants and animals and residue. 14

In the 1950, use of pesticides made food more affordable because of the abundance that could be grown. 15

Research continued in the 1970's and 80s' resulting in the greatest selling herbicide glyphosate, the low use rate sulfonylurea and imidazolinone herbicides. This time also saw the development of **triazole**, **morpholine**, **imidazole**, **pyrimidine** and **dicarboxamide** families of fungicides.16

In the 1990's, research centered on finding new members of existing families which have "greater selectivity and better environmental and toxicological profiles". Today, pest management is being achieved by genetically engineered crops designed to produce their own insecticides or exhibit resistance to a broad spectrum of herbicide products or pests. 17

My Experience

Over the past 70 years, I have witnessed and been subjected to the misuse of pesticides. Since before I can remember, the use of pesticides to eradicate insects has been common practice. However, the way in which the chemicals have been used has placed humankind at risk. The use was intended to make our lives better. Instead, the use presented a new set of problems.

In 1959, at the National Wildlife Federation 23rd Annual Convention, Dr. M. M. Hargraves addressed the issue of "Chemical Pesticides and Conservation Problems". Dr. Hargraves announced to his audience "the 'problem' of pesticides has generated considerable heat in the last few years and this largely stems from the unknown effect as yet upon human animal, aquatic and other biological values."

Dr. Hargraves further explained how mankind has adapted to his changing environment over the centuries, but we as the manipulators of inherent risks by means of new tools in our environment have a responsibility to act accordingly. He summarized the risks associated with the use of pesticides as follows:

1. *There is a loss of certain existing environmental values and ecological relationships that are displaced by the resulting new ones, and only time and readjustment will prove which we may need for survival.*
2. *There is an acquired responsibility to maintain constant surveillance or policing protection of the resulting environment since the introduction of the pesticide must now be a constant operating check in the new ecological balance established by its use.*
3. *There is a health hazard to existing individuals in the habitat, both from the effect of actual personal contact with the agent and from the need for habitat readjustment.* 18

Throughout his presentation, Dr. Hargraves presented the underlying concern about the use of pesticidal agents, arsenic, lead, sulfur, mercury, and plant glucosides such as strychnine, curare and digitalis. He further advises that petroleum and petroleum distillates are the most commonly used and oldest pesticides.

From a medical standpoint, Dr. Hargraves pointed out the implications that gasolines, fuel oils, cleaning fluids, lubricants, and solvents may be considered as pesticides. Multiple exposures inherent in petroleum and its distillation products has been shown to yield aplastic anemia, leukemia and the lymphomas in individuals who have been exposed. 19

He further explained that not all individuals react the same way to repeated exposures to pesticides, but with repeated exposures of time, susceptible individuals may develop a degree of sensitivity making the next exposure a "disastrous consequence." 20

Examples of harmful effects from exposure to pesticides resulted as follows:

Hodgkin's granuloma as a result of exposure to **Lindane**. 21

Acute and fatal aplastic anemia as a result to exposure to insecticidal powder containing **naphthalene**. 22

Leukemia has developed as a result of exposure to bug spray containing **benzene haexachloride** 23, exposure to a bug bomb 24, exposure to chlordane 25, exposure to door varnish containing petroleum distillate 26, and exposure to painting products. 27

In 1963, President John F. Kennedy requested his Science Advisory Committee review the benefits and risks of the use of pesticides in the United States. A report was generated May 15, 1963. President John F. Kennedy was concerned about our environment. The report was difficult to locate, but the following link should provide the full report.

http:/timpanogos.wordpress.com/2012/12/10/use-of-pesticides-report-of-the-presidents-science-advisory-committee-may-15-1963/

The report stated that as the need for more food became intensified, the use of pest control became necessary.

"Pesticides have made a great impact by facilitating the production and protection of food, feed, and fiber in greater quantity and quality; by improving health; and by keeping in check many kinds of nuisance insects and unwanted plants." 28

According to the report, as a result of this demand, agricultural needs entailed the largest application of pesticides in the United States. Such use reduced food losses and provided high quality foodstuffs. In turn, the productive livestock economy increased and non-food crops such as cotton, tobacco and timber also increased. 29

The adverse effect of utilizing pesticides were only discovered after a long period of time. Even in 1963, pesticides were detectable in food items, some clothing, in man and animals and in various parts of the natural surroundings. Pesticides can be carried from one locality to another by air currents, water runoff or living organisms and have persisted for long periods of time.

The report further advises that pesticides are designed to kill or metabolically upset some living target organism. The long reaching effects concluding that "pesticides constitute only one facet of the general problem of environmental pollution." 30

As of June 1962, almost 500 compounds incorporated in more than 54,000 formulations were registered for use in the United States. 31

According to the report, in 1940 the use of pesticides worldwide increased with the development of DDT and other chlorinated hydrocarbons. 32 It was further reported that over 350 million pounds of insecticides were used in the United States in 1962. An estimated 90 million acres were affected composed of farmlands, forests, and insect-breeding areas as well as wetlands. 33

As the application of pesticides increased, the study found the presence of pesticides at great distances from the place of application. Residues of **DDT** were detected in the major rivers, in ground water, in fish from fresh waters, in migratory birds, in wild animals and in shellfish. [34]

As noted, pesticides can enter the body by ingestion, absorption through skin intact and inhalation. [35]

The Panel review evidence that before pesticides are recommended for registration, considerable research was conducted as to their effects on foods, what safeguard procedures were in place to minimize risk to the consumer. At the time of the report, it was determined that residue levels were low and rarely above the legal tolerance limits. [36]

Studies show that wide use of **DDT** for Dutch elm disease control resulted in 80 percent mortalities among birds in areas heavily treated with **DDT**. [37]

President Kenney stated in the Advisory report that, "Man's primary concerns have always been the struggle for survival and improvement of his lot. As his numbers increased, he attained greater ability to manipulate his environment.

In the process he sometimes inflicted damage on himself and on his surroundings. Advances have always entailed a degree of risk which society must weigh and either accept, or reject, as the price of material progress."

The use of pesticides was both a benefit and a detriment. The material standard of living had been greatly enhanced during the 20th century by increased control over the environment

BENEFITS

According to Section II of the report, the use of pesticides has facilitated the production and protection of food, feed, and fiber in greater quantity and quality; by improving health; and by keeping in check many kinds of nuisance insects and unwanted plants. Agricultural needs have entailed the largest applications of pesticides in this country.

"Productivity has been so increased that famine is an unknown experience to the people of the developed nations. Mechanization, improved fertilizers, and the breeding of productive and disease-resistant crops have also contributed importantly. In addition, pesticides have made possible the economical production of many crops which otherwise would be available only to a limited number of wealthy consumers. ..." While reducing food losses, pest control has also resulted in foodstuffs of the highest quality."

"Besides enabling spectacular increases in agricultural production, pesticides have freed man from communicable diseases to an unprecedented extent. Furthermore, reservoirs of disease in animals, and insects which can transmit them, will remain with us for the predictable future both in this country and in other parts of the world, thus requiring a continued effort to control them."

HAZARDS

"Evidence of increasing environmental contamination by pesticide chemicals has generated concern which is no longer limited to citizens of affected areas or members of special-interest groups. During two decades of intensive technical and industrial advancement we have dispersed a huge volume of synthetic compounds, both intentionally and inadvertently. Many, such as detergents, industrial wastes, and pesticides, are now found far from the point of initial dispersal.

"Today, pesticides are detectable in many food items, in some clothing, in man and animals, and in various parts of our natural surroundings. Carried from one locality to another by air currents, water runoff, or living organisms (either directly or indirectly through extended food chains), pesticides have traveled great distances and some of them have persisted for long periods of time. Although they remain in small quantities, their variety, toxicity, and persistence are affecting biological systems in nature and may eventually affect human health. The benefits of these substances are apparent. We are now beginning to evaluate some of their less obvious effects and potential risks." 38

Chapter Six
Flame Retardants

In 1959, I initially attempted to protect our children. The only one who listened was Dr. J. B. Askew, Public Health Director for San Diego. His letter to me and those from the city schools did no good!

The article in the San Diego Union, March 19, 1979 entitled *The Dilemma – Safety or Poison, Pesticides: In the World Around Us* depicted me sitting on a flame-retardant free couch. The article appeared 20 years after my family and I were poisoned. I could not get near the flame retardant furniture because I was so severely poisoned by all chemicals. Doing so made me sick.

In the article, it explained how dangerous flame retardants are. Yet, they bring a newborn home from the hospital in flame retardant pajamas, put the baby on a flame retardant treated mattress in case there is a fire. The cure is worse than the disease.

Not too long ago, Dr. Oz had a father holding is 2-year-old son. We were told the boy was severely ill because of the flame retardant that he had been exposed to. Dr. Oz and his generation are looking for the truth. I was there before any of them were born so I know the truth. That's what all these young doctors are telling you, The Truth, no more medical secrets to make money! California and now many other states require flame retardant in all furniture.

Mona McMinn and Pauline Menzel both have colon cancer. Would they have had colon cancer if these chemical companies hadn't sprayed the schools, the food, and everything else with carcinogenic pesticides? That is the question.

Chapter Seven
Agent Orange

According to the reports, most of the veterans of Vietnam were exposed to 19 million gallons of **Agent Orange**. The use of **Agent Orange** was to reduce the foliage of the jungles so our troops could fight the enemy. Exposure to this chemical has cost the lives of many brave military men who survived the war only to be confronted with a new battle for good health years later. 40

When these veteran's complained of feeling sick after being sprayed with **Agent Orange**, they then were told, it was all in their heads. That sounds familiar! Did Dr. Edmund Keeney, Director of Scripps world famous clinic send me to his Chief of Psychiatry, Dr. Frederick Ziegler who told me it was all in my head, and I had a "phobia," and I should just go home and forget the whole thing.

So I went back to my very polluted house which the chemical company failed to decontaminate and prayed that I wouldn't have a convulsion because the muscular twitching became more violent every time I got near my polluted furniture so completely filled with **DDT** just as my body fat was! I was just a "brainless" nurse.

What about the 11 schoolgirls who were having violent muscular twitching in their classroom in New York? Erin Brockovich and her whole team were digging around outside the school because they thought that a train had spilled some toxic substance outside of the school. No way. They were poisoned in their own classroom. There is no doubt in this human guinea pig's mind!

Chapter Eight
Crib Death
Related To Pesticide Poisoning

Much mystery still surrounds the subject of "crib deaths," but several interesting pathological findings were noted under "Abnormal Parathyroids.

Here again we find the problem of calcium imbalance, but this time in pregnant women. Could this calcium imbalance in pregnant women be due to pesticides as it is in the case of the thin-shelled pelican and falcon eggs? Is the lack of the parathyroid gland or impairment of the gland in the crib death babies, as Dr. Geertinger's research indicated, also a result of faulty calcium metabolism resulting from exposure to pesticides? This question seems important since the parathyroid glands have an effect on calcium and phosphorous metabolism.

Many eminent authorities have given their reasons for believing that pesticides can cause leukemia and other forms of cancer. This brings to mind a series of articles in *Life Magazine* that were done several years ago. The articles state that extensive tests were being conducted on houses in which several members of the same family had died of leukemia or other forms of cancer.

Some of the questions raised were: Is cancer hereditary? Are there some deadly virus affecting people in these houses? Along with these questions we might also ask: Was the house fumigated with a so-called "harmless" pesticide or was it treated by putting a deadly insecticide in the attic and an even more deadly insecticide under the foundation of the house to remain there forever for the occupants to inhale?

It is contrary to logic to expect poisons to kill bugs without having an effect on people. If it can kill one living cell (plant, animal, or human), it must be insidiously doing its damage on all living cells. People as well as bugs in these houses may very well be poisoned, but since the body weight of a person is so many times greater than that of a bug, the person is poisoned more slowly.

This is why, as Dr. Pottenger stated, many people are suffering from chronic insecticide poisoning and neither they, nor their doctors, are aware of it. If these same researchers rechecked these houses again and this time looked for poisons instead of viruses, they might possibly find some startling answers.

Along this same line of thinking, we might recall a very unique and well publicized occurrence at a zoo several years ago. If you recall, several bears in the same cage died of cancer of the liver. The reasons for their deaths remain a mystery. The cages were, according to the newspaper accounts "cleaned exceptionally well."

Several more bears were put in the same cage and they too died of cancer of the liver. My question is, what exceptional methods were used to clean these cages? Were petroleum distillates used? Were the cages sprayed with insecticides? Are bears animals that lick their surroundings more than other animals?

Now that we know that these poisons are not as harmless as we are led to believe, we must go back and try to evaluate the extent of the damage we have done. We might begin by looking in our grocery stores at the many shelves full of poisons people use to poison themselves with. If we walk down the aisle we can notice that we will smell moth crystals and roach cakes that are frequently alongside baby foods and cereals.

Notice the fly strips that contain **organic phosphates**. There are usually many cardboard boxes of these and several unwrapped ones at the top of the display rack. These are guaranteed to last for ninety days and can kill flies at a distance of twelve feet even though the fly doesn't touch one. They are advertised as being so powerful that they are called "The Exterminator."

I wonder how much of this permeates into the food and how much goes into the food when the store is periodically sprayed. The Director of Public Health in San Diego states that these fly strips are not to be used in food handling establishments. Yet, they are at the top of the display rack in many stores as well as hanging in donut shops and other food handling establishments?

Well, if they didn't get you kids, they at least got the fish and the birds. Remember the mysterious fish kills and bird kills. Not a mystery to me or to Dr. Purvis Martin. He was a bird watcher and a friend of Dr. Joseph Jell, curator of birds for the Museum of Man here in San Diego.

Dr. Martin asked me to take the paper I wrote, *I Am a **DDT** Cripple* up to the top floor of the Museum of Man, which I did. What a shock. There was Dr. Joseph Jell in his white doctor's coat and the entire top floor of the Museum of Man had crates and crates of Pelican eggs and the yolk was running out of each egg. Dr. Jell said it was impossible to get one egg to hatch because the **DDT** had taken the calcium out of all of the pelican eggs just as the **DDT** had taken the calcium out of my 4-year-old son's femur after he slept in the house with a 50 percent concentration of what pest control company claimed was harmless white powder.

Many children played at my house and were continually breathing this **DDT** powder into their lungs just as my whole family did. My family became acutely ill from constant exposure to the **DDT**.

As I said before, the only person who knew that I was telling the truth was Dr. J. B. Askew, Public Health Director of San Diego. Each time I ran into the poison, I called Dr. Askew since I now had a "Hot Line" to him. Every time I called he personally answered the phone.

That article was written by Dr. Askew after I called him and told him that a woman grocery store checker who was 8 months pregnant had a shelf at her check stand with a huge display of these fly strips on her counter. These were wrapped in cardboard boxes and her counter area reeked of this pesticide that this pregnant mother breathed in during her 8-hour shift.

Where was OSHA? Weren't they supposed to provide safety in work places? I had the grocery store manager remove the dangerous fly killers from the check-out counters and called Dr. Askew. That's when he issued the warning on, "Fly Killers Use". Remember, on September 2, 1964, I was the one that complained about schools being sprayed with repeated doses of poisons and Dr. Askew, our wonderful Public Health Director listened.

No one but Dr. Askew would even take the poisoning of you children seriously except all the doctors that did all the research before many of you were born. That's why I call this multi-generational poisoning a type of genocide.

Did you see the children convulsing when Saddam Hussein poisoned his people with whatever poisons he used? Is this all right in your crazy world? It's not okay with me, the human guinea pig!

Another time, an uninformed housewife, me, went grocery shopping at our main grocery store called White Front. My groceries included two beautiful heads of lettuce. I put all the supposedly safe groceries in my car and immediately knew I was in trouble when I suddenly developed blurred vision and got out of the car to vomit. There was a strange smell that reeked from my grocery bag. I picked up the two heads of lettuce and threw them away.

By now I was acutely ill and was hoping that a policeman would come by and I would ask him to drive me home. But no such luck. When I stopped trembling, I drove myself home to my much polluted house.

I called Dr. Askew and he answered my "Hot Line" call. A week later, an article appeared in the San Diego Union stating no more **lindane** vaporizers were in San Diego. Oh, well. The heck with everyone else in the country, it's okay. To have a **lindane** vaporizer spray on all the beautiful produce just in case the crop dusters missed a big, bad bug.

All my beautiful mothers got pregnant just as God had planned. Now, we have to have "Invitro Fertilization!" Well, as I always said, God's beautiful world was just great. We loved God's plan. Now we have some scientist trying to upstage God that's why the world has gone to hell in a hand basket.

Not only is this great research, he quotes actual patients that have become ill or died after as little as one exposure. This research was February 27, 1959.

As I said to the Nurses' Health Study, *My research is Better than Yours.*

October 24, 1977

Mrs. Geraldine Fiedler
San Diego, California

Dear Mrs. Fiedler,

Please find enclosed a copy of the final report of analysis on the fabric submitted to our laboratory. As we discussed, in our telephone conversation, the limits of our laboratory instrumentation did not allow the fine definition required to adequately evaluate the potential contamination. Our selection of West Coast Technical was based upon a quality history of work by them.

If I can be of further assistance or service to you please do not hesitate in contacting me. It is my hope this analysis helps to further direct your activities in maintaining a healthful environment for yourself.

Sincerely,
- S -
Kenneth S. Cohen
Industrial Hygienist / Toxicologist

On October 24, 1977, I received the above letter and report from Dr. Kenneth Cohen on a piece of velvet material that had been sent to his Reference Center Laboratories for testing. The report shocked even Dr. Cohen who is an Industrial Hygienist /Toxicologist. There was so much and so many kinds of pesticides that filled all the beautiful fabrics in Mr. Walter Broderick's Design Center.

As I said in my newspaper article, I had hired one of Mr. Broderick's interior decorators. She told me that she was "allergic" to fabrics in his store. His fabrics were as polluted as my house and furniture and why should they be? We pay pest control companies to routinely spray our homes and businesses, so actually we pay them to poison us. How stupid can we be!

Dr. Kenneth Cohen, an honest toxicologist asked me to speak at his seminar at Scripps La Jolla when he gave his seminar on Toxins. This was about 25 years ago.

At that time, he said that people were using about 300 pesticides in their homes and gardens thinking that they were "harmless." Ironically, my grandson's mother-in-law is in charge of the nursing program at Scripps La Jolla.

So then how did I lose the case against a local pest control company when I sued them for poisoning my family? Well, I had doctors who were ex-military doctors of World War II who were told that DDT was safe. Didn't they de-louse their pilots when they landed after transporting planes from one country to another as they did my friend, Hal Hunt, as you read earlier? Both Ardath and Hal were graduates of Berkeley and lovely friends. Hal died of Alzheimer's disease and Ardath died of heart problems.

So why did I lose the case when I sued the pest control company? I brought the lawsuit not for the money, but because of how everyone and everything was being poisoned. It was a moral obligation and part of my commitment to God to protect God's children.

Well, the truth of the matter is, I was one very sick poisoned woman fighting a multi-billion dollar chemical empire. Let me truthfully say that I was easily shot down by the pest control company's powerful lawyer who shortly after he won the case became a judge.

The jury had never heard of pesticide poisoning. One old jurist slept throughout the whole trial! The judge thought I was a nut case, especially after UCLA sent their expert witness.

All that against me, one dumb R.N! Well, the expert witness mumbled something about maybe it was the petroleum distillate that made our family ill. I lost the case that cost me thousands of dollars.

The **DDT** that injured my 4-year-old son who limped on a leg brace for a year and a half, was having totally white stools and this formally healthy boy that his pediatrician, Dr. Lawrence Reck, describes as a little football player, was now pale and looked very ill, which he was. So, as I said, we lost the case.

Let me quote Dr. Francis M. Pottenger, Jr., MD of Monrovia, California, who was doing research on pesticides and helped Rachel Carson write, *The Silent Spring,* and was the consultant for Adele Davis.

March 13, 1962

Dear Mrs. Fiedler:

It was good of you to let me know how your trial came out. I sincerely regret that you lost, for your illness was, indeed, real. I knew the toxicologist well and was surprised that he proved not to be my friend.

I shall tender no bill for my appearance, since it proved of no avail to you. Please tell Attorney Stutz (my lawyer) that I appreciate his kindness to Mrs. Pottenger and me.

I trust that your health continues to improve. We shall always be glad to hear from you.

With regards to you and Mr. Fiedler, I am,

Sincerely yours,
-S-
Francis M. Pottenger Jr. M.D.

In 1966, a friend called me to tell me that *Learning to Live with Poisons* (not how to stop using them) program was to be presented by the San Diego Chapter, American Society of Safety Engineers at a National Poison Prevention Week Symposium. It was to be held on March 24, 1966, at the Islandia Hotel here in San Diego.

Well, you can bet I would attend this symposium to hear all the cooperating agencies: San Diego Department of Public Health, Children's Hospital of Los Angeles, University of California at Los Angeles, Academy of Pediatrics, Automobile Club of Southern California, California State Department of Public Health. Impressive, wouldn't you say! After all the research since 1945, here come the big wheels!

Welcoming remarks were given my old friend Dr. J. B. Askew, M.D. M.P.H., Director Dept of Public Health, County of San Diego. "Poison Information-

Overview" was presented by Mrs. Claire Barton R.N., Chief Poison Information Center, Children's Hospital of Los Angeles. "Pesticides and their Hazards" was presented by the expert witness who testified against me at my trial.

Well, here was that same expert witness with this huge lighted screen telling of the great danger of all the hazardous pesticides. He was contradicting his earlier testimony. What a surprise!

So when he was in the midst of all his vast knowledge which he was so proud to tell everyone, I stood up and loudly said, "Do you remember when you testified in court that you thought that it was the petroleum distillates that was making my family ill? You didn't offer to let your family sleep in a bedroom full of a commercial concentration of 50 percent of "harmless **DDT**" which almost killed us did you?"

He stuttered for at least a half a second, but came up with more of his magnificent excuse! "Do unto others as thou would have others do unto you!" Aren't doctors great and nurses nothing!"

After lunch Dr. Irma West, California State Department of Public Health, Berkeley, gave her presentation *Poisons and the Child*. Dr. Irma West and Dr. Francis Pottenger worked together.

Well, no one ever said let's get rid of all these useless (dangerous) poisons except me! That's right! It was just my phobia as Dr. Frederick Ziegler called it!

Well, kids, I hope you are convinced by now that, it was okay to spray you kids in school since no one believed Dr. Pottenger and Dr. Purvis Marten, Dr. Morton Biskind's famous research, or Dr. Nan Kathryn's truths! Nope, I hope you learn to live with poisons (and the damage they cause to life in our country).

When I walk around Overlook Heights where I have lived since 1950, I am saddened because all my friends are dead from the original group that lived here. I feel like crying when I see those that moved up here 10 years after. These human wrecks that were vibrant, healthy neighbors have Alzheimer's and look like walking dead!

I have finally been able to write this book to warn you about pesticides because I was deadly ill from our forced air system taking a commercial concentration of 50 percent **DDT** throughout our house even though the directions read, "Never, never, never use this inside a house, only under the house or in an attic!"

Well, doctor, your erroneous words convinced a jury and judge who had never heard of pesticide poisoning and it was that testimony that caused me to lose my case. When I lost, all the babies that I promised God that I would work to save went out the window.

My family went through hell, and I never had another baby because I didn't want 95 percent of my DDT to go to a baby, as Dr. Pottenger said it would.

Dr. Pottenger did my second fat biopsy a year after the first fat biopsy. The first one showed I had 33 parts per million of **DDT** in my body fat. A year later the second biopsy showed that I had more **DDT** which constituted 45 parts per million of **DDT** in my body fat.

Dr. Pottenger said that the attempt to decontaminate our house had failed miserably and we must move out, which we did in 1960. This was just as the woman physician did in "The Fumigation Chamber" article. Even though she was a doctor, they treated her as "brainless" like me, "The Spray Lady".

I did not want to drive from San Diego all the way to Dr. Pottenger's clinic in Monrovia, California, so I asked my guardian angel, Dr. Purvis Martin, my mentor, to take out the stitches of the second fat biopsy, which he generously did. He also talked to Dr. Pottenger and was told the whole story of how serious this poisoning was.

After that is when I received a letter from Dr Purvis Martin dated July 17, 1969. In his letter he said he had read, *I am a DDT Cripple* and made some suggested editing and then said that I should "send a copy to his cousin, Mary Harrington Hall. She would like very much to interview you and develop this into a magazine article, this should be in a national publication."

Dr. Purvis Martin knew what they were doing and that's why when he performed my hysterectomy in 1969, he sent the book *The Silent Spring* and told me to read it and to write a paper, that we did resulting in *I Am a* ***DDT*** *Cripple*.

Dr. Martin chose that title, and he wanted his cousin, editor of *Psychology Today* to publish our paper in a national magazine. I'm sorry to say, Mary Harrington Hall died, so the article was never published.

I was desperately trying to protect my thousands of Mercy babies and the whole generation of Baby Boomers and their babies. A *Prevention Magazine* article states that traces of insecticides were present in the blood of 93 percent of pregnant women. Another article said pesticides were present in 83 percent of the baby's umbilical cords.

Prevention Magazine, April 2012, featured an article that said all the people that have been poisoned just like my family had been and who could have been spared the hell the pest control and chemical companies caused which I believe was all for money, damn money!

Dr. Martin talked to Dr. Francis Pottenger who was doing research on pesticides. He came into court and testified for me because he saw the danger to all of you and your unborn children being poisoned.

His testimony when he told the court that the best way for me to get rid of the **DDT** in my body was to have a baby and 95 percent of the poison would go to the baby and if I nursed the baby 100 percent of the poison would go to the baby! **That's what I call multi-generational poisoning!**

After I had been so severely poisoned, I took my 7-year-old daughter to school where I learned later they were spraying two water trucks of poison on you kids! I ran into the school nurse and screamed, "They're poisoning the kids! She said, "I agree with you, but I need this job!" Insanity!

I went to the Education Center 5 times and begged them not to poison the kids and they laughed and called me the "spray lady". To no avail!

Then I stood up at the P.T.A. meeting and said, "I am a registered nurse and I work at Mercy Hospital where every doctor and nurse must account for every drop of medicine.

However, when it comes to pesticides and herbicides, the maintenance crew who were spraying the kids, the teachers and the entire staff of the schools.

They not only sprayed the kids in school, they sprayed the Little League fields, children's playgrounds and parks. They used weed killer everywhere.

Do you spray the same amount of poison on a 40-pound child as you do on a 200-pound teacher?" Soon the teachers were asking me to stop the poisoning!

In 1960, I saw a **lindane** vaporizer that sprayed the produce in White Front, our main grocery store.

Today, Dr. Oz is shocked to learn that there is pesticides in food, arsenic in apple juice, and mercury in fish. According to Dr. Oz on his show, he's worried about his children and grandchildren.

Conclusion

I am back to square one. In 1959, when I was poisoned with a commercial concentration of 50 percent **DDT**, which was blown throughout my home by a forced air heating system, my family and I, and possessions were exposed to poisonous **DDT**.

The directions on the package clearly stated, this product was NEVER to be used inside of a house. It was only to be used under the house or in an attic. Did the pest control operator care? His job was to get rid of the bugs not worry about me.

This is what happens to you when you pay a pest control company to fill your home with poisons that will make you sick or even kill you. You have read about all the people that have gotten sick or died because the pest control companies have lied to you. They have said that these chemicals are non-poisonous. Lies, Lies, Lies. The research in my book proves this.

On April 19, 2015, on *Sixty Minutes*, Scott Pelley did an exposé on how inhumane Asada Harinsuit was when he poisoned his own people in the Middle East. Our own chemical companies are doing that very thing to all of you and you are paying them to be poisoned and even thanking them.

The chemical companies were so nice when they poisoned you in the 50s' and 60s' as little children. As early as 1959, I was fighting to stop the spraying because I realized how deadly those poisons are. Take it from me. Being poisoned was hell. You never fully recover from being poisoned because the original poison damages your entire body.

Ask the veterans who so valiantly served their country and were exposed to Agent Orange and bug bombs that were supposed to be safe and were deadly! Anyone who has been poisoned can tell you it is hell.

As Collen Murphy, spokeswoman for Sharp Hospital said, "If you want the truth, ask a nurse." Having been a nurse for 70 years, I heard and know the truth.

In 1959, I wrote to CBS and told them my story. Dan Rather was the anchorman then. However, since the entire country was brainwashed by the lying chemical companies, Dan Rather, the doctors, my jury, no one listened. I am not blaming anyone.

The only other person who really knows the truth is my lawyer, Sidney Stutz. When I was deathly ill, he was so kind to drive me to my physician Dr. Francis

M. Pottenger in Monrovia, California. He saved my life. I underwent treatment with Dr. Pottenger for 3 years. He had also saved the life of my friend Hal Hunt, a pilot who was also exposed to **DDT**. Every time he landed is military plane, he and the plane were deloused.

No one listened to Secretary of the Interior Stewart Udall who correctly called the practice, "peopleocides". No one listened to Dr. Pottenger who in 1960 said, "Man will pollute himself out of existence." Samuel Geddes said the same thing. Could they have been right?

I learned from Dr. Pottenger in 1960 about a book being written that would "rock the nation." The book became *The Silent Spring* by Racheal Carson. Carson's work published the research of Dr. Pottenger to make the public aware of the toxic chemicals in our society.

In 1969, after Dr. Martin did my hysterectomy, he sent me a copy to Mercy Hospital of *The Silent Spring* encouraged me to read it and write a paper about my experience. This book is finally coming out over 50 years later.

Dr. Pottenger also assisted Adele Davis in writing her healthy eating publications. Dr. Oz says, *Get Health Back*. His classmate, Dr. Joel Furhman, has written many books on how to eat correctly. I know I have heard this before. Wasn't that what my mother taught me, the Mediterranean diet?

Did I tell you that I have been part of the famous most quoted Nurse's Health Study since its inception 38 years ago? Did I tell you that when I grew up, all food was organic? My mother and I had a restaurant and we grew our own food. We did not need to look for organic food. All food was organic, just as God made it.

Many of the doctors today like Dr. Nicholas Perricone, Dr. Stephen Sinatra, and Dr. Victor Marchione are telling you how to eat correctly like my mother taught me.

As the voice of experience, I wrote the Nurse's Health Study to tell them about my research. My generation was the best. People helped one another. Today's generation appears to have digressed. Who has destroyed this country?

Laura Bush knows the score. Her top priority as first lady was to get the first ladies all over the world to protect women and children. Children are gifts from God and don't ever forget it.

In 1943, a priest told me at Mercy Hospital that this country will be destroyed by the downfall of the family unit. Truer words were never spoken!

When big money put the Sisters of Mercy out of business, San Diego lost the goose that laid the golden egg. My "Angles of Mercy" are no longer.

Gone are the good old days when a patient walked through the doors of Mercy Hospital and they knew God's angels would be there to assist them no matter what.

I went back to playing bridge at M.C.R.D. where I play with another fellow nurse cadet named Brandi Costello. Nicki O'Leary is 90 years old and she and I worked in the defense plants when they were short of help and we were known as "Rosie the Riveter". We were part of the "greatest generation" on earth.

These nurses worked hard to bring care to their patients. The training is different today. The one-on-one care is replaced with computer terminals. It is difficult to accept what this nursing profession has become.

You were right, Tom Brokaw, mine was the best generation society ever produced and everyone knows it. That is why I also dedicate this book to the greatest people on earth the Mothers and Fathers.

As the Ten Commandments says, "Honor thy Mother and thy Father." I survived to share my story. Take heed. God knows and has the last say in all things.

Pesticides, Chemicals, and Poisons Used In United States

Agent Orange
Aldrin
Anesthetics
Arsenic
Bacillus Thuringlensis
Benzo(a)pryene
Bisphenol
BPA
Bominated Flame Retardants
Carbonate Pesticides
Carbon Monoxide
Carcinogen
Chlordane
Chlordane
Chlorinated Hydrocarbon
Chloromethyl-Methyl ether CMME
Chlorpyrifos (CY)
Cholinesterase Inhibitors
Cyanide gas
Cyfluthrin
DBCP
DDT
DDT and Seven
DDVP
DI toluene dilsocyanate
Diazinon
Dibrom

Dieldrin
Dioxin
Drin changes to Dieldrin
Dursban
EDB
Endosulfan
Endrin
Ficam
Fire Retardant
Fyrol
Genetically Modified Organisms (GMO)
Halogenated Hydrocarbon Anesthesa
Heavy Metal
Heptachlor
Heptachlor Expoxide
Herbicide Paraquat
Hydrocardon
Hydron cyanide gasses
Lawncare chemicals
Lead
Lindane
Lycopene
Malathion
Maneb
Methoxychlor
Methyl Carbamates
Methyl Parathion
Mirex
Monoethyl Phthalate (MEP)
Moth balls

Moth Flakes
Mutagen
Naphthalene
Nitrogen dioxide
Non-GMO
OrganicPhosphate Insecticides
Organochloine Pesticides
Organophosphates
Orthene
Oxychlordane
Parthion
PCBs, or polychlorinated biphenylate
Peopleocides
Perfluorinated chemicals
Perthane
Petrocemical Hypersensitivity
Petrochemical
Petroleum distillates
Phosdrin
Phthalate DEHP
Polyurethane Foam
Polyurethane
Ploy-vinyl chloride Pyrethroid Insecticides
Pyrophus
Pryothrum
Rotenone
Ryanic
Sulfur dioxide
Systox
TEEP

Tiodan
Toxaphene
Toxins
Triclosan
TRIS

Footnotes

1. Oz, Dr. Mehmet, *Eat to Live* Forward.

2. Ibid.

3. Fuchs, Nan Kathryn Fuchs, PHD, Editor-in-Chief, *Women's Health Letter. The 456 Most Powerful Healing Secrets.*

4. Carson, Rachel, *The Silent Spring*, pg. 197.

5. Carson, Rachel, *The Silent Spring*, pg. 172.

6. Carson, Rachel, *The Silent Spring*, pg. 212.

7. Unsworth, John, *History of Pesticide Use* May 10, 2010, citing Impetus for sowing and the beginning of agriculture: Ground collecting of wild cereals. M.E. Kislev E. Weiss and A. Hartmann, Proceedings of the national Academy of Sciences. 101 (ppgs. 2692-2694) (2004)**http://www.weizmann.ac.ll/kimmel-arch/od/17_Kislev2004.pdf**

8. Unsworth, John, *History of Pesticide Use* May 10, 2010, citing Primal SeedsOrigin of Agriculture. **http://www.primalseeds.orgl/agricult.htm**.

9. Unsworth, John, *History of Pesticide Use* May 10, 2010, citing *The History of Pesticides, Organic Pesticides,* September 19, 2008. http://www.blog.ecosmart.com/index.php/2008/09/19/the-history-of-pesticides/.

10. Unsworth, John, *History of Pesticide Use* May 10, 2010, citing Janek, J., History of *Horticulture, Roman Agricultural History,* Purdue University. http//www.hort.purdue.edu/news/cro/Hort_306/text/lec18.pdf.

11. Unsworth, John, *History of Pesticide Use* May 10, 2010, citing Smith, A.E. and Secoy D. M., *Forerunners of Pesticides in Classical Greece and Rome,* J. Ag. Food Chem. 23 (6) 1050 (1975). http://www.hort.purdue.edu/newscrop/history/lecture18/r_18-1.html.

12. Unsworth, John, *History of Pesticide Use* May 10, 2010, citing, *The History of Pesticides, Organic Pesticides,* September 19, 2008. http://www.blog.ecosmart.com/index.php/2008/09/19/the-history-of-pesticides/.

13. Unsworth, John, *History of Pesticide Use* May 10, 2010, citing Delaplane, K.S., Pesticide Usage in the United State: History, Benefits, Risks, and

trends; Bulletin 1121, November 2000, Cooperative Extension Service, The University of Georgia College of Agricultural and Environmental Sciences.

http//pubs.cases.uga.edu/casespubs/pubs/PDF/B1121.pdf.

14. Unsworth, John, *History of Pesticide Use* May 10, 2010, citing, *The History of Pesticides, Organic Pesticides,* September 19, 2008. http://www.blog.ecosmart.com/index.php/2008/09/19/the-history-of-pesticides/.

15. Unsworth, John, *History of Pesticide Use* May 10, 2010, citing Delaplane, K.S., Pesticide Usage in the United State: History, Benefits, Risks, and trends; Bulletin 1121, November 2000, Cooperative Extension Service, The University of Georgia College of Agricultural and EnvironmentalSciences. http//pubs.cases.uga.edu/casespubs/pubs/PDF/B1121.pdf.

16. Unsworth, John, *History of Pesticide Use* May 10, 2010, citing Wessles Living History Farm, York Nebraska: Farming in the 1950s & 60s. **http://www.living** historyfarm.org/faminginthe50s/pests_08.html .

17. Unsworth, John, *History of Pesticide Use* May 10, 2010.

18. Unsworth, John, *History of Pesticide Use* May 10, 2010.

19. Hargraves, Dr. M. M., "Chemical Pesticides and Conservation Problems", Feb 27, 1959 23rd Annual Convention of the National Wildlife Federation New York pg. 2.

20. Hargraves, Dr. M. M., "Chemical Pesticides and Conservation Problems", Feb 27, 1959 23rd Annual Convention of the National Wildlife Federation New York pg. 3.

21. Hargraves, Dr. M. M., "Chemical Pesticides and Conservation Problems", Feb 27, 1959 23rd Annual Convention of the National Wildlife Federation New York pg. 4.

22. Hargraves, Dr. M. M., "Chemical Pesticides and Conservation Problems", Feb 27, 1959 23rd Annual Convention of the National Wildlife Federation New York pg. 6.

23. Ibid.

24. Ibid.

25.Ibid.

26.Ibid.

27.Ibid.

28.Ibid.

29.The President's Science Advisory committee, "Use of Pesticides" May 15, 1063 Washington D.C. pg. 2.

30.The President's Science Advisory committee, "Use of Pesticides" May 15, 1063 Washington D.C. pg. 3.

31.The President's Science Advisory committee, "Use of Pesticides" May 15, 1063 Washington D.C. pg. 3-4.

32.The President's Science Advisory committee, "Use of Pesticides" May 15, 1063 Washington D.C. pg. 5.

33.Ibid.

34.Ibid

35.Ibid. pg. 6.

36.Ibid.

37.Ibid.

38.Ibid. pg. 8

39.Ibid.

40.**http://www.history.com/topics/vietnam-war/agent-orange**.

The following article, "The Problem with Pesticides," by *Toxics Action Center* will introduce you to the world of Pesticides.
http://www.toxicsaction.org/problems-and-solutions/pesticides

Science Advisory Committee Report to review the benefits and risks of the use of pesticides in the United States generated May 15, 1963.

http://timpanogos.wordpress.com/2012/12/10/use-of-pesticides-report-of-the-presidents-science-advisory-committee-may-15-1963/

Bibliography

Perricone, Dr. Nicholas, *Eat To Live*, citing Oz, Dr. Mehmet, Forward in *Eat to Live*.

Fuchs, Ph.D., Nan Kathryn, *The 456 Most Powerful Healing Secrets*.

Pesticides: In The World Around Us, San Diego Union Tribune, March
19, 1979.

UC Scientists Believe Tris May Cause Sterility In Boys, San Diego Union, August 8, 1977.

Toxic Chemicals May Lower Sperm Density, San Diego Union, September 14, 1979.

Egge, Rose, *Local Doctors Link Pesticides To Infertility In Women*, November 5, 2013. **http://www.komonews.com/news/health/Local-doctors-link-pesticides-to-infertility-in-women-230694311.html**

Cancer Was No Factor, Only Toxicity Inspired Flammability Standards,Copley News Service, 1979.

Roueche, Berton, *The Fumigation Chamber*, Annals Of Medicine, January 4, 1988.

Letter from Herbert G. Klein, The San Diego Union, October 10, 1967

Letter from Mrs. Louise S. Dyer, President, Board of Education

Letter to Health Chairman, Skyline Council, Parent & Teacher Association, August 16, 1965

Agent Orange
http://www.history.com/topics/vietnam-war/agent-orange

Hunt, H.C., *My Experience with Insecticides,* April 13, 1963.

Hunt, B.A., M.A., Ardath, *Protect Yourself from Chemical Poisoning,*
Bestways, June 1978.

Biskind, M.D., Morton S, Quote from *Public Health Aspects of the New Insecticides,* November 1953, Page 331.
http://link.springer.com/article/10.1007%2FBF02883493 - page-1

Chlordane, Environmental Protection Agency (EPA), Hazard Summary - Created in April 1992; Revised in January 2000.
http://www.epa.gov/ttnatw01/hlthef/chlordan.html

Biskind, M.D., Morton S Public Health Aspects of the New Insecticides,
Amer. Jour. Dig, Dis., November 1953, pg. 331.

Fielder, Geraldine, *I Am A DDT Cripple.*

Quote from an article by Dr. Abraham B. Bergman, regarding "crib deaths"

Quote about "Abnormal Parathyroids".

A Nightmare In Niagara, Long Buried Chemicals Rise Up To Scarify A Neighborhood, Time Magazine, August 14, 1978.

Udall, Stewart L., *A Frank Report from the Secretary of the Interior,* True, the Man's Magazine, August 1965.

Hargraves, Dr. M.M., *Chemical Pesticides and Conservation Problems,* The Mayo Clinic, Rochester, Minnesota.

Use Of Pesticides, President's Report of Science Advisory Committee, May 15 1963. **http://www.jfklibrary.org/Asset-Viewer/Archives/JFKPOF-087-003.aspx**

EPA Tests Find Pesticides In Nursing Mother's Milk, San Diego Union regarding a study in 1975

Mother's Milk or Mother's Poison? Pesticides in Breast Milk."
http://eap.mcgill.ca/MagRack/JPR/JPR_07.htm

Pesticide Traces Found in Babies, New York Times News Service,
October 1968.

Larynx Spasm Blamed In 10,000 Baby Deaths, October 25, 1968.

Researcher Has New Crib Death Theory, San Diego Union Tribune,
April 5, 1979.

Link Seen to Smog, Sudden Infant Death, San Diego Union Tribune,
October 1979.

Suit Claims Pesticide Made 7 Children Ill, San Diego Union Tribune, Thursday, October 19, 1979.

Dana, Margaret, *Residue in Mothballed Baby Clothes, Can Be Highly Toxic to Infants,* San Diego Union Tribune, Thursday, April 11, 1968.

Obstetricians Issue Warning on Chemicals, The San Diego Union Tribune, September 24, 2013.

Insecticide Mystery, Poison In Rhine Destroys Fish, San Diego Union Tribune, June 25, 1969.

Warning Issued on Fly-Killers' Use, San Diego Union Tribune, June 25, 1969.

Poison Mystery is Created by Hit-and-Miss Insecticide, by The San Diego Union's Science Writer.

Allchin, Dr. Douglas, Rachel Carson & Silent Spring, Chapter 17, Doing Biology. **http://www1.umn.edu/ships/db/carson.pdf**

Bed Bug Pesticide Poisoning' Killed California Woman And Six Other Tourists In Thailand, By Daily Mail Reporter, Updated: 11:18 EST, 10 May 2011.

Cox, Caroline, *Cyfluthrin Fact Sheet,* Fluoride Action Network Pesticide Project, Published in Journal of Pesticide Reform/Summer 1994, Vol. 14, No. 2. **http://fluoridealert.org/wp-content/pesticides/cyfluthrin.facts.1994.htm**

Chlorpyrifos, Pesticide Action Network, North America. **http://www.panna.org/resources/chlorpyrifos**

Doyle, Kathryn, *Study Links Pesticide Exposure In Pregnancy To Autism,* NEW YORK Monday, June 23, 2014 8:37am EDT. **http://www.reuters.com/article/2014/06/23/us-pesticides-pregnancy-autism-idUSKBN0EY1BF20140623**

Konkel, Lindsey, Staff writer, *Autism Risk Higher Near Pesticide-Treated Fields, Study Says,* Environmental Health News, June 23, 2014.

California Pesticide Initiative, Committee for Biological Pest Control in Agriculture, October 16, 1989.

Fikes, Bradley J., *Parkinson's Tied To Pesticide Parkinson's: Brain Mutation And Exposure Makes People More Susceptible,* San Diego Union Tribune, November 28, 2013.

Fuchs, Ph.D., Nan Kathryn, *Slow Death By Rubber Duck,* Journal of Natural Healing.

BPA-Free Plastics Are Safe, Right? Don't be so sure..., *What you*
need to know to protect yourself, by Dr. Nan Kathryn Fuchs, Journal of
Natural Healing, April 2014.

Letter from Kenneth S. Cohen, Industrial Hygienist, followed by a copy of the final report, West Coast Technical Service, Inc. fabric sample.

West Coast Technical Service, Inc, fabric sample report.

The Allergy Explosion: Are Chemicals to Blame? "Ten thousand Americans are allergic to the Twentieth Century." Bestways, June 1978.

Letter from Dr. Francis M. Pottenger Jr. M.D., March 13, 1962.

Learning to Live with Poisons, San Diego Chapter, American Society of Safety Engineers, National Poison Prevention Week, March 24, 1966.

Casper Won't Spray His Shots, It Reminds Him of Insecticide, The San Diego Union, Sports Editor, June 11, 1969.

Williams, Dr. David, *Insecticides and Autoimmune Diseases, Alternatives for the Health Conscious Individual,* March 2010.

GAO says picture-perfect lawn might pose a hazard to health, The San Diego Union, March 29, 1990.

The Truth About Cats, Dogs & Lawn Chemicals, The History of Lawn Chemicals, Pesticide Watch Education Fund, July 2008.

Hofman, Janet, *Flea Spraying Blamed, Illnesses Force Her to Move,* Oceanside Blade-Tribune, 1976.

As Nature Made Them, Prevention 2012

Whitehead, Dean, *Facts And Myths About Petroleum Distillates;*
http://www.protectall.com/artpetdist.aspx

Glyphosate, Pathways to Modern Diseases II: Celiac Sprue and Gluten Intolerance, Toxicology 2013

Beamish, Rita, *Nurse Practitioners Seek Bigger Role*
Your AARP
California News, April 2012

Wallis, David, *The Late Shift: Second Acts in Nursing, See why these 4 people switched careers to care for others* AARP Bulletin, June 2014. **http://www.aarp.org/work/working-after-retirement/info-2014/ second-career-in-nursing.2.html**

Unsworth, John, *History of Pesticide Use,* May 10, 2010.

Additional References

Agency for Toxic Substances and Disease Registry (ATSDR). *Toxicological Profile for Chlordane* (Update). Public Health Service, U.S. Department of Health and Human Services, Atlanta, GA. 1994.

U.S. Environmental Protection Agency. ***Deposition of Air Pollutants to the Great Waters. First Report to Congress***.EPA-453/R-93-055. Office of Air Quality Planning and Standards, Research Triangle Park, NC. 1994.

U.S. Environmental Protection Agency. ***Toxicological Review of Chlordane (Technical).*** *In Support of Summary Information on the Integrated Risk Information System (IRIS).* National Center for Environmental Assessment, Office of Research and Development, Washington, DC. 1997.

U.S. Department of Health and Human Services. Registry of Toxic Effects of Chemical Substances (RTECS, online database). National Toxicology Information Program, National Library of Medicine, Bethesda, MD. 1993.

U.S. Department of Health and Human Services. Hazardous Substances Databank (**HSDB, online database**). National Toxicology Information Program, National Library of Medicine, Bethesda, MD. 1993.

U.S. Environmental Protection Agency. *Updated Health Effects Assessment for Chlordane.* Environmental Criteria and Assessment Office, Office of Health and Environmental Assessment, Office of Research and Development, Cincinnati, OH. 1988.

U.S. Environmental Protection Agency. ***Integrated Risk Information System (IRIS) on Chlordane***. National Center for Environmental Assessment, Office of Research and Development, Washington, DC. 1999.
Occupational Safety and Health Administration (OSHA). Occupational Safety and Health Standards, Toxic and Hazardous Substances. *Code of Federal Regulations*. 29 CFR 1910.1000. 1998.

American Conference of Governmental Industrial Hygienists (ACGIH). *1999 TLVs and BEIs. Threshold Limit Values for Chemical Substances and Physical Agents. Biological Exposure Indices*. Cincinnati, OH. 1999.

National Institute for Occupational Safety and Health (NIOSH). ***Pocket Guide to Chemical Hazards***. U.S. Department of Health and Human Services, Public Health Service, Centers for Disease Control and Prevention. Cincinnati, OH. 1997.

Helfetz, Ruth M. and Taylor Sharon S. "Mother's Milk or Mother's Poison? Pesticides in Breast Milk: Journal of Pesticide Reform. Vol. 9, No. 3, Fall 1989.

Calabrese, E.J. 1982 Human breast milk contamination in the United States and Canada by chlorinated dydrocarbon insecticides and industrial pollutants: Current Statue. J. of Amer. Coll of Toxicology. 1(3).

Bradbury, S.P. and J.R. Coats. 1989. Comparative toxicology of the pyrethroid insecticides. Rev. Environ. Cont. Toxicol. 108.

U.S. EPA. Office of Pesticides and Toxic Substances. Office of Pesticide Programs. 1987. Pesticide fact sheet: Cyfluthrin. No. 164. Washington, D.C. (December 30.)

Farm Chemicals '92. 1992. Willoughby, OH: Meister Publishing Company.

California Dept. of Pesticide Regulation. Information Services Branch. 1993. Summary of pesticide use report data: Annual 1991. Indexed by chemical. Sacramento, CA (January 25.)

U.S. Dept. of Agriculture. National Agricultural Statistics Service. Agricultural Statistics Board. 1994. Agricultural chemical usage: 1993 field crops summary. Washington, D.C.: (March).

U.S. Dept. of Agriculture. National Agricultural Statistics Service. Agricultural Statistics Board. 1992. Agricultural chemical usage: 1991 fruit and nuts summary. Washington, D.C.: (June).

Whitmore, R.W., J.E. Kelly, and P.L. Reading. 1992. National home and garden pesticide use survey: Final report, Volume 1. Executive summary, results, and recommendations. Research Triangle Park, NC: Research
Triangle Institute.

Cremlyn, R.J. 1991. Agrochemicals: Preparation and mode of action. Chichester, U.K.: John Wiley & Sons.

Corbett, J.R., K.W. Wright, and A.C. Baillie. 1984. The biochemical mode of action of pesticides. Second edition. London, U.K.: Academic Press.

U.S. EPA. Office of Pesticides and Toxic Substances. 1986. The review of toxicology data in support of the registration of Baythroid 240 ornamental pyrethroid insecticide Tempo 2. Memo from J.E. Whalan, Hazard Evaluation Division, to George LaRocca, Registration Division. Washington, D.C. (August 18.)

Al-Rajhi, D.H. 1990. Properties of Ca+2 + Mg2 - ATPase from rat brain and its inhibition by pyrethroids. Pest. Biochem. Physiol. 37:116-120.

Ramadan, A.A. et al. 1988. Action of pyrethroids on GABA receptor function. Pest. Biochem. Physiol. 32:97-105.

Ramadan, A.A. et al. 1988. Actions of pyrethroids on the peripheral benzodiazepine receptor. Pest. Biochem. Physiol. 32:106-113.

Morgan, D.P. 1989. Recognition and management of pesticide poisonings. Washington, D.C.: U.S. EPA. Office of Pesticide Programs. Health Effects Division.

U.S. EPA. Office of Pesticide Programs. 1989. "Tox one-liners": Cyfluthrin. Washington, D.C. (June 28.)

Wadleigh, R.W. et al. 1991. Effect of temperature on the toxicities of ten pyrethroids to German cockroach. (Dictyoptera: Blattellidae). J. Econ. Entomol. 84(5):1433-1436.

Pauluhn, J., et al. 1988. Methodological aspects of the determination of the acute inhalation toxicity of spray-can ingredients. J. Appl. Toxicol. 8(6):431-437.

U.S. EPA. Office of Pesticides and Toxic Substances. 1987. Review of acute toxicology data in support of the registration of Tempo 20% Wettable Powder for use in food handling establishments. Memo from J.E.

Whalan, Hazard Evaluation Division, to George LaRocca, Registration Division. Washington, D.C. (February 24.)

Miles Inc. Agriculture Division. 1991. Material Safety Data Sheet: Tempo 2EC. Kansas City, MO. (January 30.)

Eil, C. and B.C. Nisula. 1990. The binding properties of pyrethroids to human skin fibroblast androgen receptors and to sex hormone binding globulin. J. Steroid Biochem. 35(3/4):409-414.

U.S. Dept. of Health and Human Services. Public Health Service. 1991. Sixth annual report on carcinogens. Summary. Research Triangle Park: National Institute of Environmental Health Sciences.

U.S. Dept. of Health and Human Services. Public Health Service. Agency for Toxic Substances and Disease Registry. 1993. Toxicological profile for xylenes. (October.)

U.S. Dept. of Health and Human Services. Public Health Service. Agency for Toxic Substances and Disease Registry. 1990. Toxicological profile for ethylbenzene. (November.)

Noble, R.M. and D.J. Hamilton. 1985. Stability of cypermethrin and cyfluthrin on wheat and storage. Pestic. Sci. 16:179-185.

Dicke, W., H.-D. Ocker, and H.-P. Thier. 1988. Rckstandsanalyze von pyrethroid-insecticiden in getreide, mahlerzeugnissen und brot. Z. Lebensm. Unters Forsch 186:125-129.

McEwen, F.L. 1986. Residues of synthetic pyrethroid insecticides on horticultural crops. Pestic. Sci. 17:150-154.

CRC Press. 1991. EPA lists 14 more pesticides linked to possibly faulty data. Pesticide & Toxic Chemical News (August 7): 8-9.

U.S. EPA. Communications, Education, and Public Affairs. 1993. Craven Laboratories case concludes with guilty pleas for falsifying pesticide tests. Press Advisory. Washington, D.C. (December 17.)

U.S. EPA. Communications, Education, and Public Affairs. 1994. Craven Laboratories, owner, and 14 employees sentenced for falsifying pesticide tests. Press Advisory. Washington, D.C. (March 4.)

Shehata, A.F., et al. 1987. Some factors influencing persistence, hydrolysis, downward movement and leachability of cyfluthrin in Egyptian soils. Annals Agric. Sci. (Fac. Agric., Ain Shams Univ., Cairo, Egypt) 32(3):1677-1687.

Class, T.J. and J. Kintrup. 1991. Pyrethroids as household insecticides: analysis, indoor exposure and persistence. Fresenius J. Anal. Chem. 340:446-453.

Stout, D.M., C.G. Wright, and R.B. Leidy. The determination of cyfluthrin in air and on surfaces. Abs. Papers Amer. Chem. Soc. 207: AGRO #36.

U.S. EPA. Office of Pesticides and Toxic Substances. 1987. Registration of Tempo* 2 (containing cyfluthrin) and risk assessment of pest control officer (PCO) use in buildings. Memo from J.E. Whalan, Hazard Evaluation Division, to G. LaRocca, Registration Division. Washington, D.C. (August 27.)

U.S. EPA. Office of Pesticides and Toxic Substances. 1987. Revised risk assessment of pest control officer (PCO) use of Tempo* 2 insecticide in buildings. Memo from J.E. Whalan, Hazard Evaluation Division, to G. LaRocca, Registration Division. Washington, D.C. (November 10.)

Laughlin, J., K. Newburn, and R.E. Gold. 1991. Pyrethroid insecticides and formulations as factors in residues remaining in apparel fabrics after laundering. Bull. Environ. Cont. Toxicol. 47:355-361.

Nelson, C. et al. 1992. Laundering as decontamination of apparel fabrics: Residues of pesticides from six chemical classes. Arch. Environ. Contam. Toxicol. 23:85-90.

U.S. EPA. Office of Pesticide Programs. Ecological Effects Branch. 1989. EEB review: Proposed $18 for use on pears and interplanted apples. Washington, D.C. (January 30.)

Estesen, B.J. et al. 1992. Residual life and toxicity to honey bees (Hymenoptera: Apidae) of selected insecticides applied to cotton in Arizona. J. Econ. Entomol. 85(3):700-709.

Taylor, K.S., Waller, G.D., and L.A. Crowder. 1987. Impairment of a classical conditioned response of the honey bee (Apis mellifera L.) by sublethal doses of synthetic pyrethroid insecticides. Apidologie 18(3):243-
252.

Terry, L.A., D.A. Potter, and P. Spicer. 1993. Insecticides affect predatory arthropods and predation on Japanese beetle (Coleoptera: Scarabaeidae) eggs and fall armyworm (Lepidoptera: Noctuidae) pupae in
turfgrass. J. Econ. Entomol.:872-877.

U.S. EPA. Office of Prevention, Pesticides and Toxic Substances. 1992. Completion of the review of cyfluthrin mesocosm study. Memo from D.J. Urban, Environmental Fate and Effects Division, to G. LaRocca,
Registration Division. Washington, D.C. (July 29.)

Mokry, L.E. and K.D. Hoaglund. 1990. Acute toxicities of five synthetic pyrethroid insecticides to Daphnia magna and Ceriodaphnia dubia. Environ. Toxicol. Chem. 9:1045-1051.

Georghiou, G.P. 1990. Overview of insect resistance. In Green, M.B., H.M. LeBaron, and W.K. Moberg (eds.). Managing resistance to agrochemicals: >From fundamental research to practical strategies. p. 18-41. ACS Symposium Series #421.

Marshall, D.B. and D.J. Pree. 1986. Effects of pyrethroid insecticides on eggs and larvae of resistant and susceptible populations of spotted tentiform leafminer. Can. Ent. 118:1123-1130.

Lagadic, L. et al. 1993. Pharmokinetics of cyfluthrin in Spodoptera littoralis (Boisd.). I. In vivo distribution and elimination of [14C] cyfluthrin in susceptible and pyrethroid-resistant larvae. Pest. Biochem. Physiol. 45:105-115.

Reidy, G.F., et al. 1990. Increased glutathione s-transferase activity and glutathione content in an insecticide-resistant strain of Tribolium castaneum (Herbst). Pest. Biochem. Physiol. 36:269-276.

Atkinson, T.H. et al. 1991. Pyrethroid resistance and synergism in a field strain of the German cockroach (Dictyoptera: Blatellidae). J. Econ. Entomol. 84(4):1247-1250.

Cochran, D.G. 1991. Extended selections for pyrethroid resistance in the German cockroach

(Dictyoptera: Blattellidae). J. Econ. Entomol. 84(5):1412-1416.

Kerns, D.L. and M.J. Gaylor. 1992. Insecticide resistance in field populations of the cotton aphid (Homoptera: Aphididae). J. Econ. Entomol. 85(1):1-8.

Martinez-Carrillo, J.L., L.P. Schouest, Jr., and T.A. Miller. 1991. Responses of populations of the tobacco budworm (Lepidoptera: Noctuidae) from northwest Mexico to pyrethroids. J. Econ. Entomol. 84(2):363-366.

Lemke, L.A., P.G. Koehler, and R.S. Patterson. 1989. Susceptibility of the cat flea (Siphonaptera: Pulicidae) to pyrethroids. J. Econ. Entomol. 82(3):839-841.

Mobay Corporation. Agricultural Chemicals Division. 1991. Material Safety Data Sheet: Baythroid 2. Kansas City, MO.

Miles Inc. Agriculture Division. 1991. Material Safety Data Sheet: Tempo 20% Wettable Powder. Kansas City, MO. (January 30.)

Sittig, M. 1991. Handbook of toxic and hazardous chemicals and carcinogens. 3rd Edition. Park Ridge, NJ: Noyes Publications. v.2 p.1161-1162.

Made in the USA
Monee, IL
04 November 2026

67381839R00089